What People Are Saying About
The Perfect Formula Diet

The Perfect Formula Diet is a wonderful book—I had the good fortune to review each chapter as it was written and adapt my eating plan to its principles. The research is so thorough and its practices have worked for me. Now, in over 520 days of my day to day approach to healthful eating and with over 50 pounds of weight loss, I feel great. After many years of diets, weight loss and re-gain, I believe I'm now have a long-term approach to healthful eating.

— KATHY STERNBACH, M.ED, M.B.A, BEHAVIORAL HEALTH CONSULTANT

Janice Stanger writes a powerful testimony to the health value of a plant-based diet. She not only cites the supporting evidence for her claims but in many cases intelligently uses metaphors that illustrate her points. It's a great read, both for the public and for the professional. I wholeheartedly endorse it.

— T. COLIN CAMPBELL, PH.D., AUTHOR *THE CHINA STUDY*

I can't recommend most diet books because small errors in interpretation of the scientific literature can result in devastating diseases for some people. If you want to read on that gets it right, Dr. Stanger's *The Perfect Formula Diet* can help people reduce their risk of chronic disease and lead a more healthful and pleasurable life.

— JOEL FUHRMAN, M.D., CO-FOUNDER OF EAT RIGHT AMERICA
AND AUTHOR *EAT TO LIVE*

Reading this book, I was very impressed! It covers so many different aspects of why we need to eat whole foods exclusively, and is backed up with all the latest research! Get this book in everybody's hands! Bravo for a wonderful effort!

— RUTH HEIDRICH, PH.D., IRONMAN TRIATHLETE AND
AUTHOR *A RACE FOR LIFE, CHEF*, AND *SENIOR FITNESS*

Dr. Stanger makes eating well and regaining lost health easy to understand in *The Perfect Formula Diet*. She sticks right with the facts. Her efforts to provide exhaustive scientific research for her book offer a formidable challenge to all naysayers.

— JOHN McDOUGALL, M.D., FOUNDER OF THE McDOUGALL PROGRAM
AND AUTHOR *THE McDOUGALL PROGRAM FOR WOMEN*
AND *THE McDOUGALL PROGRAM FOR MAXIMUM WEIGHT LOSS*

The Perfect Formula Diet is a must read for anyone who loves to eat and wants to lose weight. Dr. Stanger offers an extremely intelligent science-based, practical guide for transitioning to a whole-food eating plan. You *can* put an end to compulsive food cravings, yo-yo dieting and poor health and this book will show you how. And you'll be saving the planet at the same time! This book will be required reading for my clients.

— JULIE M. SIMON, M.A, M.B.A, M.F.T, PSYCHOTHERAPIST
AND EATING DISORDER SPECIALIST

This diet is simple and effective, the science is irrefutable. This is the most important book you will read regarding your health and your family's health. The writing is a joy to read; the message is a must read.

— ANDY LAUB, FOUNDER OF FARMERS MARKET TEA

The Perfect Formula Diet explains the science, appreciates the art, and captures the magic of whole foods.

— REX BOWLBY, AUTHOR *PLANT ROOTS*

In her book, Dr. Stanger shares her journey from illness to perfect health, empowering all who read *The Perfect Formula Diet*. This book is a perfect tool for teaching future generations how to live a lean, green, and inspired life.

— BARBARA GATES, DIRECTOR OF LEAN AND GREEN SCHOOLS

THE PERFECT FORMULA DIET

How to Lose Weight and Get Healthy *Now*
with Six Kinds of Whole Foods

Janice Stanger, Ph.D.

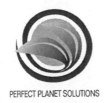

PERFECT PLANET SOLUTIONS

San Diego, California

Copyrighted Material

The Perfect Formula Diet
How to Lose Weight and Get Healthy Now with Six Kinds of Whole Foods

Copyright © 2009 by Janice Stanger, Ph.D.

ALL RIGHTS RESERVED WORLDWIDE

No part of this publication may be reproduced, stored in a retrieval system or transmitted, in any form or by any means—electronic, mechanical, photocopying, recording or otherwise—without prior written permission from the author, except for the inclusion of brief quotations in a review or for research purposes.

For information about this title or to order other books and/or electronic media, contact the publisher:

Perfect Planet Solutions
5580 La Jolla Blvd. #459
La Jolla, CA 92037

www.perfectformuladiet.com

Library of Congress Control Number: 2009906534
ISBN: 978-0-9841067-3-8
Printed in the United States of America

"Our body is a machine for living.
It is organized for that, it is its nature."
~ Leo Tolstoy

"Facts do not cease to exist because they are ignored."
~ Aldous Huxley

Contents

Preface: Perfect Odyssey ix

Chapter 1: Perfect Body. 1

Chapter 2: Perfect Weight 11

Chapter 3: Perfect Foods 23

Chapter 4: Perfect Protein. 31

Chapter 5: Perfect Nutrients 47

Chapter 6: Perfect Formula Diet. 59

Chapter 7: Perfect Rotation 71

Chapter 8: Perfect Start 97

Chapter 9: Perfect Logistics. 113

Chapter 10: Perfect Price. 127

Chapter 11: Perfect Evidence. 131

Chapter 12: Perfect Health 145

Chapter 13: Perfect Defenses. 153

Chapter 14: Perfect Balance. 169

Chapter 15: Perfect Puzzle Completed. 181

Chapter 16: Perfect Planet. 199

Chapter 17: Perfect Home 209

Chapter 18: Perfect Next Steps 219

Chapter 19: Perfect Climate 229

Chapter 20: Perfect Story. 239

Chapter 21: Perfect Resources. 243

References 253

Index 255

DISCLAIMER

This book contains general information about health and nutrition and is not meant to substitute for medical care, treatment, or advice from a health care professional. If you believe that you, your child, or any other person whom you care for has a health problem, the author and publisher strongly recommend that you obtain the services of a physician or other appropriate health care professional.

The statements in this book have not been evaluated by the FDA, and as such, shall not be construed as medical advice, implied or otherwise. This book is not intended to diagnose, treat, cure, or prevent any disease. Information in this book is intended to be and should be used for educational purposes only.

If you, your child, or any other person whom you care for has a health problem you should always consult with a physician before making dietary changes.

Under no circumstances should you, your child, or any other person whom you care for change the dosage or timing of or discontinue any prescription or non-prescription medication that person is using, except under the supervision of and with the consent of a qualified, licensed health care professional.

Reference to specific people, groups, or products in this book does not mean that the author or publisher endorses these entities or that these entities endorse this book.

This book is not intended to be a textbook covering all research in nutrition and health. Considerable effort has been devoted to making this book as accurate as possible. However, there may be typographical errors or other mistakes. This book should therefore be used as a general guide for informed decision making and not as your only source of information on nutrition and health.

You are urged to consult the references and other resources used for this book, as well as conduct supplementary research, and to keep an open, critical, and questioning mind in learning about weight, nutrition, and health. Think about where research is published, who did it, who paid for it, and whether the findings are consistent with other studies, human history, common sense, and your own experience and observations.

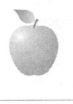

Perfect Odyssey

Natural Perfection

Your body is a complex marvel of intricate design, with everything you need to be lean, healthy, and energetic already built in. Don't let anyone tell you that you're irreparably overweight, sick, or otherwise "flawed." *You are already naturally perfect.*

The secret—so simple yet so profound—of permanent weight loss and ageless health is to work *with* your body instead of against it. By going with this natural flow, you'll slide to your preferred weight as effortlessly as a plant grows toward the sun.

You have likely been hurt by harmful diets that don't work, that raise and then smash your dreams, leaving you in worse shape than when you started. I want you to succeed with a new, effective set of choices. Throughout this book, I'll be talking with you and sharing what I learned the hard way.

Once I was trapped in the muddle of chronic overweight, multiple health problems, and hopeless distain for my body. Assisted by my daughters and pioneering researchers, I struggled to Perfect Health and a trim figure.

I want to share the breakthrough formula I discovered with you and see you marvel at the same transformation to the health, youthful energy, and lean weight you desire and deserve. You shouldn't suffer one day longer than you have to! You don't need to put up with being overweight or obese for years to come!

In the past, you based your diet on information you had at the time. With 21ˢᵗ century knowledge, you are free to make better choices. After all, what will your life be like in 10 years if you don't find a better way to eat and stay healthy now?

I appreciate your confidence in me, and will earn it by sharing hard-to-get information about whole foods that has been hiding in plain sight.

Living To Eat

The story of food is the story of my life. Food was a family obsession. As far back as I can remember, my days centered around meals and snacks. Special events were inseparable from extraordinary meals. The highest compliment for anyone in my family was praise that a meal they cooked or hosted was "delicious."

I was always planning what to eat next. Amazingly, I was thin—almost skinny—during my growth years in Philadelphia. I had been tall for my age as a child, but stalled at 5 feet 4 inches at age 12. After that, I gained a few pounds and, although still an appropriate size, became obsessed with weight.

I tried different crazy diets popular in the 1960s. Like most kids in my generation, I was indoctrinated early in the supposed importance of "protein." My favorite food was meat, and I could easily devour a pound of steak, half a chicken, or an entire slab of ribs at one meal.

So it's no surprise I ended up on the animal-based Stillman Diet, the precursor to subsequent "high protein" diets. How clever I thought it was to eat the hamburger and leave the bun. Little did I dream then that several decades later the fallacy of this eating plan would become overwhelming for me.

A Bag Of Cookies, Graham Crackers, And Three Chocolate Bars

The turning point in my ability to control my eating came in the summer between my junior and senior years of high school. I won an award to attend a summer science program in Wisconsin. Feeling isolated from the other students, I took refuge in food—ice cream to be more specific. I began to eat two or three scoops a day, with a side of whatever other junk foods I could dig up the money for.

When I returned home in the fall, I began to eat secretly and obsessively. Any binge eater will understand the cycle. I was disgusted with myself and my growing weight, so I comforted myself with massive amounts of foods such as graham crackers, ice cream, cookies, cake, and candy. A typical eating episode might include a bag of cookies, graham crackers, and three chocolate bars.

However, the eating worked emotionally only if no one else saw it. Since I lived at home and had little money, this limited the number of binges. My weight went from 116 to 128 pounds, which was heavy for my tiny frame but still far from obese.

Once away at college, things went from bad to worse. At least at home we always had vegetables, fresh fruit, and salad. In the college eating halls, the offerings were skimpy and not too appetizing. Except for their banana bread. I began to eat huge amounts of it as well as binge on other junk foods just about every night.

Before I knew what had happened, my weight skyrocketed to 165 and beyond. After 165, I stopped weighing myself, so I can't tell you how much higher it went. To make the situation worse, I had little money for clothes and no fashion sense. I always wore ill-fitting clothes that made me look even heavier than I was.

My obsession with weight and obsession with food fed each other, and my life was totally out of control. Binge eating reduced my stress level, but only temporarily. Then my weight gain and self-disgust fed into a mountain of sadness and despair.

Depression ruled my days. Once I was walking across campus and suddenly felt so hopeless that I sank to the ground and sat there for hours staring into space until a kind student I didn't even know spoke to me in a caring voice and led me back to my dorm.

California Dreaming

After college I hadn't the foggiest clue what I wanted to do. An acquaintance was driving to San Francisco to visit family and invited me along on what was intended to be a quick cross-country road trip.

I'll never forget my first glimpse of the hills of San Francisco. After growing up in flat suburbs, the rise and fall of the streets were profoundly beautiful and mysterious. People smiled. I instantly fell in love with the city and decided to stay. The Bay Area was my home for the next 27 years.

A funny thing happened when we hit San Francisco. My binge eating simply evaporated. A couple of times, out of habit, I tried to down a bag of cookies and a quart of ice cream, but could never eat more than a fraction of the targeted food. So to save money, I stopped buying the binge junk food. Still, although my weight stabilized, it did not decrease until a cross-country road trip several years later when my boyfriend and I didn't have money and were forced into calorie restriction.

My Adulthood Was Not A Health Model

The aim of this Preface is to give you the story of how the Perfect Formula Diet came to be, so I'll stay focused on weight and health with the bare outline of other milestones. Since I loved learning and going to school, I earned an MBA from UC Berkeley and a Ph.D. in Human Development and Aging from UC San Francisco. I got married at 28, had two daughters when I was 30 and 32, and separated from my husband when our kids were only three and five.

Through all of this, my weight fluctuated and averaged about 145 for many years. Overwhelming fatigue and low energy topped my health care issues. I fell asleep on the bus to work, nodded off in my office, and fought drowsiness on long drives.

Since I had been heavily exposed to tobacco smoke as a child, my respiratory system was my weak link. I suffered from chronic sinus, ear, and bronchial infections. Another painful problem was a burning tongue and mouth. No doctor or dentist could ever tell me the cause. Severe endometriosis and near constant depression—despite taking antidepressants—also made my life miserable.

Intense but sporadic headaches haunted my adult life, as well. I lived in fear of these agonizing episodes, which had no discernable cause. When I hit my forties, the headaches morphed into daily trials. The first thing I did *every* morning was roll out of bed and race to the bathroom for over-the-counter painkillers to allow me to get through the day.

Amazingly, I accepted my weight and health issues. After all, didn't everyone have problems? Physicians seemed relatively unconcerned and were of little or no help, except to prescribe antibiotics for the sinus infections (which always came back). Going to the doctor and taking pills were a normal part of my life. And just about everyone I knew was on a diet or planning the next weight loss attempt.

Out Of The Food Trap

Luckily for me, my strong-willed daughters put me on the road to my Perfect Weight and glowing health. My 13 year old declared she would no longer eat meat, poultry, or fish, and her 11 year old sister followed her lead a couple of weeks later.

I was horrified and convinced my offspring would suffer dangerous malnutrition. After all, I had been raised to believe meat was the premier food, packed with nutrients and the center of any decent meal. My first reaction was to persuade the kids to eat meat and get off their self-imposed diet. Both my children have a strong oppositional-defiant streak, so that strategy backfired big time.

Defeated, but biding my time, in 1995 I began my research into nutrition that continues to this day. Being well trained in methodology in graduate school, I searched out medical textbooks, prestigious medical journals, physicians, dieticians, and other nutrition researchers. To my total amazement, I learned that people who avoided animal foods were healthier than other people.

The rest of this book shares the secrets learned from analyzing more than a thousand studies and observing what happens when you adopt a whole foods diet.

My energy level is now intense, I no longer fall asleep except at night (and then I sleep soundly), and I haven't had a sinus, bronchial, or ear infection or burning tongue or mouth since starting my current diet. Headaches are exceptionally rare. Best of all, depression and food cravings are distant memories.

At age 57 I'm at my Perfect Weight and in Perfect Health. I take no prescription or over-the-counter meds. I don't have allergies, arthritis, skin problems, digestive problems, circulatory or heart problems, liver, kidney, or gall bladder problems or any eye or autoimmune diseases. I don't have diabetes or cancer and my cholesterol is 145. My blood pressure is typically about 90 something over 60 something.

For the last 10 years or so, I've felt as if I've been aging in reverse. I'm in better health now than I was 30 years ago.

I LOVE the Perfect Formula Diet. This way of eating has taken me to a whole new level not just physically, but also emotionally and spiritually. How often do you hear anyone talk about loving a diet?

Thanks To The Pioneers Of Nutrition Evolution

Dr. Neal Barnard, Dr. John McDougall, Dr. Joel Fuhrman, Dr. Michael Greger, T. Colin Campbell, Ph.D., Dr. Dean Ornish, and other trailblazers whose research and writings leave no doubt about the desirability of a whole-foods diet are an inspiration to all seekers of health. This book builds on and aims to weave together their critical discoveries. Any errors in the process of synthesizing information are mine alone.

Just as important are the numerous leading-edge cooks whose satisfying recipes, generously shared, make a whole-foods diet the tastiest and most appealing on the planet.

I am so grateful for the training from the University of California San Francisco program in Human Development and Aging and my nurturing professors. The requirements to earn my Ph.D. provided a foundation for understanding human health and choices.

Even more importantly, my teachers focused on how to distinguish good research from bad, learn to be critical and question experts, weigh controversial issues, and recognize bias and weak conclusions. These skills and my insatiable curiosity enable me to plow through apparently conflicting studies until I get to the bottom of what's really going on. The University of California San Diego medical library has been my second home for many years.

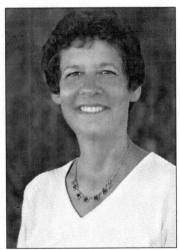

My editor, Andrea Glass, has worked with me tirelessly and patiently.

This book presents 14 years of solid research, critical thinking, and exploration. Enjoy, question, and draw your own conclusions on this remarkable journey.

This book would still be just an idea without the love and encouragement of my family and friends. May you thrive in Perfect Health.

Janice Stanger, Ph.D.

CHAPTER 1

Perfect Body

You get only one body for your lifetime, so it's lucky for you that your body is naturally perfect. Your physical self is an awesome composition of 100 trillion cells, all orchestrated to keep you vigorous and at your ideal weight well into your nineties, or older.

You have good reason to be proud of yourself, even if you want to make some changes. Your body knows how to heal cuts and bruises, digest food, use oxygen, get rid of wastes, pump blood, fight off microbes, rebuild damaged cells, and turn sound waves into understandable speech—all without your conscious control.

Your body in its wisdom also knows how to keep you at a trim weight. This book teaches you a system to work *with* your body so you achieve all the weight and health benefits of following nature's plan.

Working With Your Naturally Perfect Body

Losing weight is a matter of getting out of nature's way by eating the food your body is designed to thrive on. Have you ever seen an overweight coyote, fox, squirrel, rabbit, mountain lion, or deer in the wild? No, and you never will. Your body is built to naturally stay as lean as a wild animal's.

While your body is inherently perfect in its design, you may be challenged by unnatural conditions that push the limits of what you can handle. Symptoms of disease and ballooning waistlines are not "mistakes." Instead, your body is doing everything in its power to counter the damaging conditions it must survive in our current era of manufactured foods and a chemical-laced environment. You are probably also harmed by a serious deficiency of nutrients found only in whole foods.

If you have chronic pain or illness or have suffered a heart attack or stroke, you may feel your body is betraying you. Yet your body wants to achieve glowing health. Are you letting yourself down through poor decisions and second-best nutrition? Are you accelerating your own aging instead of fostering lifelong high functioning? You *can* learn—and enjoy—nature's eating plan to take your health in a new direction.

On your usual diet, you may sense of loss of control—a frightening feeling that there's nothing you can do to make things right with yourself. On the Perfect Formula Diet, you regain a firm grip on moving in a healthy direction. You do have it in your power, through some simple choices, to achieve youthful energy, enviable health, an attractive weight, a positive outlook, and the ability to take charge of your eating and your lifestyle.

On previous weight loss diets, you may have glumly subsisted on tiny, microwaved meals with 300 or so calories compressed into way too few bites of food. Maybe you tried to fill up on a side salad that was large in volume but seemed to strangely shrink once it hit your stomach. The Perfect Formula Diet encourages you to sit down and eat an entire plateful of satisfying food. Eat until you are no longer hungry, and when you are hungry, eat again.

On the Perfect Formula Diet, you snack as a way to avoid overeating at meals. In fact, you'll move away from the concept of "meals" and let your hunger guide when you should fuel your body.

Your Body—Your Best Partner

When you choose to work with your body to give it everything it needs, while not overwhelming it with damaging substances or more than is optimal, you'll naturally flow to your Perfect Weight and stay there effortlessly. Perhaps you have given up on healthy eating because you think you lack "willpower." But willpower is needed only when you are fighting your body—for example, by holding your breath.

When you are working with, and not against, your body, no willpower is required because your naturally Perfect Body is designed to be happy when you're giving it what it needs. Think of how easy and pleasant it feels if you sleep when you're tired, breathe when you need a breath, or sip cool water when you're thirsty.

Doesn't following most diets feel like walking, running, or riding a bike uphill into the wind? You get tired and frustrated because you're not working *with* your body—and that takes as much energy as going against gravity. Setting yourself against the powerful forces of nature is a surefire recipe for failure in the long-run and often even in the short-run.

In contrast, losing weight with the Perfect Formula Diet is like rolling downhill with the wind at your back. The forces of nature work to your advantage.

Your hunger is your built-in guide to achieving this balance, so thank your body when you're hungry, and eat the Perfect Formula Diet until you're satisfied.

Getting To Know Yourself

You don't need to understand every detail of how your body is regulated (and not even the best scientist does) to appreciate how finely balanced your systems are and the damage that will result from working against your body's basic design. However, you can work with your body most powerfully when you better understand how you're put together and function. Insights about your body are the most effective basis for trusting in yourself and making informed decisions.

You have about 70,000 miles of blood vessels carrying nutrients, oxygen, and other vital necessities to every cell in your body. This awesome living highway circulates nutrients, carries away toxic wastes, brings in immune system forces for protection, and fuels metabolic processes. Each of these functions is necessary for health—indeed for life itself.

Your cells are grouped into many kinds of tissues and organs, each needing to be coordinated with all the others. Again, your body has complex mechanisms, such as your nervous system and your immune system, to make sure all parts work together flawlessly so you'll be around to see another sunrise.

Individual cells do not live as long as you do. Cells naturally die when they're worn out, diseased, or mutated. If this process, called apoptosis, does not occur when it should, illness and tumors are likely to result.

Apoptosis is a selective pruning that encourages vigorous new cells, just as pruning a rose bush clears the way for the plant's continuing growth and beauty. Your body needs to put together up to 5,000,000 cells each second to replace the cells that correctly die.

More Is Not Better For You

Your naturally Perfect Body is a finely tuned system, more complex than the most intricate machine. To stay in balance and healthy as long as possible, all your systems need to operate in defined, and usually quite narrow, ranges.

When you think about nutrition, the word "adequate" may carry the sense of not quite "enough." After all, an adequate amount of a given nutrient can appear to verge on insufficient. You may aim to eat *more* of certain substances seen as keys to good health. These include isolated vitamins, minerals, and proteins you take as an "insurance policy" to make sure you're getting plenty for optimal health.

In its innate wisdom, your body wants to maintain an ideal *balance* of vitamins, minerals, and different sources of calories—proteins, fats, and complex carbohydrates. When you eat too much of any one of these nutrients, your body's ratios are out of whack, and you "crave" the missing foods needed to counteract the excessive amounts of other foods.

This imbalance is an important force driving the "carb cravings" sensationalized by many ineffective diet books. If you eat whole foods in ideal proportions to each other, your body will automatically receive the correct amount of healthy complex carbohydrates to fuel your everyday activities and maintain your Perfect Weight. Your food cravings will melt into history.

Partnering: Make It Happen

All the 100 trillion cells in your body are interconnected in multiple ways that scientists are only starting to understand. When one part of your body is damaged by excessive or harmful substances, the chaos spreads. Gaining weight is often a noticeable consequence of this loss of balance.

So the first readjustment of your view of food is to see that the ideal amount of any given nutrient is the quantity your naturally Perfect Body needs, but not so much that you have problems resulting from more than is optimal.

Your body keeps meticulous track of nutrients, calories, rest, oxygen, water, and other survival needs. When one of these critical elements is lacking, your body will send you out to get it. Resisting your body's commands is futile in the long term, and often even in the short term. When you get too much, on the other hand, health symptoms and appetite cravings to balance out the excess will follow.

You may use "willpower" to work against your body, depriving it of what it needs or flooding it with too much, but your success will be only temporary at best. *To lose weight permanently and find robust health, you must learn to work with your body.*

Take advantage of the fact that your body precisely measures and balances essential nutrients by following the Perfect Formula Diet and learning to respect your body's signals. Honor your hunger—don't stave it off, fight it, satisfy it only partially, or ignore it.

Trust your body's call for energy and nutrients by eating Perfect Foods in balanced proportions, and soon you will be your Perfect

Weight, feeling energetic and with a second chance at youthful good health.

Effective Thinking Vs. Wishful Thinking

If you browse through shelves of diet books, you'll notice that most are look-alikes. You're instructed to eat more "servings" of fruits and vegetables, substitute whole grains for white flour and white rice a few times a day, liberally pour the olive oil, and build meals around controlled portions of "low fat" dairy products, poultry, and fish so you can get enough of that supposedly elusive nutrient called protein.

Portion control, a code word for "hunger," is fundamental for many run-of-the-mill approaches to weight loss. Or maybe you picked up a protein-obsessed hang-on from the 1960s that tells you to eat all you want, as long as it's nothing but animal foods and veggies.

The stories on nutrition research you read in popular magazines and newspapers are most often based on the "apple a day" view of health. The idea is that minor modifications to a commonplace eating pattern, such as adding one or two apples or forkfuls of broccoli each day, will somehow create a more healthful pattern of eating and lead to weight reduction.

Researchers look at one isolated aspect of overall food intake (such as fat, fiber, calcium, protein, or Vitamin C) and measure whether relatively small changes in this part of the diet will lead to measurable health or weight results.

Here's the thing. Often everyone in the nutrition studies you hear about is eating the same food with negligible variations. Researchers may then exaggerate trivial differences in diet to draw misleading conclusions.

The "apple a day" view of health fits perfectly with the theory of "superfoods," a trendy media topic. The idea of a "superfood" is akin to the idea of "Superman" but tied to nutrition. These are specific foods or nutrients that are supposed to be powerful enough to rescue you from all the ill effects of your dietary mistakes. While this is an appealing myth, a smattering of "superfoods" is no more likely to have a profound effect on your health than Superman is to swoop through the window and carry your pesky co-worker off to a desert island.

In following past diets, haven't you found the "apple a day" theory is a failure as a guide to attaining good health and achieving permanent, meaningful weight reduction? On the Perfect Formula Diet you'll follow a best-case *pattern* of eating and not focus on one food or nutrient in isolation from this pattern.

But What About Genes?

Isn't weight at least partly determined by genes? Aren't some people better off on one set of foods, while others thrive on the exact opposite diet?

Let's shine some common sense on this issue. Your genes are designed to keep you healthy and optimize survival, not to make you sick. People with seriously defective genes would not be likely to have children and pass on their genetic code. Your ancestors were survivors and you have that biological heritage.

In any case, rates of overweight, obesity, and many chronic diseases have been skyrocketing at way too rapid a rate for genetic change to be the dominant cause.

Of course every person is different from every other person genetically, unless he or she has an identical twin. But why would this mean we each should be eating radically different diets? Is this the case anywhere else in nature?

Are certain rabbits better off eating plants while others prosper on meat? Are some cows better off dining on grass, while others are designed by nature to eat nuts or fish? Will some mountain lions grow healthy on deer, while others thrive on pine bark? The idea is silly. Within any one species eating the foods that nature intended, all individuals do best on roughly the same diet, despite clear genetic differences among individuals. Why would humans be any different?

Not all genes are expressed; how your genetic code moves into action is critically determined by nutrition, chemicals you are exposed to, and other environmental factors. Think of your genes as being similar to the blueprint for a house whose actual construction depends on available material, labor, and terrain.

Studies of people who move from one country to another find that the risk of illness and obesity matches the person's *adopted* country, not their country of origin, after the person begins eating the diet of the country that he or she moved to.

The fact that migration changes the risks of disease and obesity is clear and compelling evidence of the importance of lifestyle choices and environment in determining the way your unique genes express themselves. *So don't let anyone tell you that you're doomed to obesity by faulty genetics.*

Commitment Is Everything

Just the fact you're reading this book shows you're health conscious, curious, and persistent. Use these traits to build your commitment to the best food choices.

Commitment is necessary to make the Perfect Formula Diet work for you. While willpower involves forcing yourself to do something you really don't want to do, commitment is based on the choice to stick with something you want to do even though you may have other attractive choices or options.

For example, you may commit to doing volunteer work every Wednesday after work. You could spend the time getting extra tasks done at the office instead, or talking with your friends, playing a game, or otherwise relaxing. But if you are totally committed to the volunteer work, you'll show up as promised anyway and feel good about your decision.

In the same way, following the Perfect Formula Diet requires commitment until it becomes habit. This book will reinforce your commitment with information and motivation. Commitment freely made from the heart can make any task achievable and even enjoyable.

True, you'll need to develop new habits and give your taste buds a few weeks to change. Yet, the reward for your efforts is that all of your 100 trillion cells will look and feel superb. Your health can't wait!

The Story Condensed

You've probably found that past weight loss programs had temporary success at best and were counterproductive at worst. Now you have another chance to succeed on a science-based 21st century eating plan. By working *with* your naturally Perfect Body, you can coast to the weight you want and health you deserve.

Genetics won't stand in your way, but run-of-the-mill diets will. The little-known truth is that the *ideal* amount of any nutrient is the quantity your intricate body systems need, and not so much that you're thrown off balance. On the Perfect Formula Diet, you change the pattern of what you eat so you stay full and satisfied. Simply adding an apple a day or some other superfood to an otherwise unhealthy eating plan won't do the trick.

With your desire for health, you can enjoy the Perfect Formula Diet and stay at your Perfect Weight forever. You can maintain youthful energy and functioning for decades into your adult years. As you read on, be prepared for little-known facts that will demolish nutrition myths you've been taking for granted.

Each chapter ends with a summary "The Story Condensed." If you are pressed for time, you can read this summary for an overview of key chapter points. Later, to understand all the information that supports your success, aim to read through the whole chapter.

CHAPTER 2

Perfect Weight

At your Perfect Weight, you will look your best, foster robust health, and recharge your energy. But here's the best news. You will maintain this weight effortlessly as long as you follow the Perfect Formula Diet. You can reach and stay at your Perfect Weight more easily than you think.

Traditional Diets Don't Work (Duh)

A headline-grabbing Harvard study proves beyond any doubt that traditional diets don't work. This research measured how four common diets achieved weight loss over a two year period.

The prescribed meal plans were all based on limited amounts of eggs, milk, meat, olive oil, vegetables, fruits, nuts, and whole grains—too little total food to satisfy most adults. Researchers aimed to adjust the amount of fat and protein in each diet by small variations in the relative proportion of each food.

For example, one of the diets called for a six inch banana while another prescribed an eight inch banana. How often have you seen fellow shoppers stalking the produce section looking for exactly the right size banana? If you see anyone putting a tape measure to a banana, you can guess that person is participating in a silly government-funded diet study wasting your tax dollars.

You are probably not surprised to learn that few study participants followed their assigned diet and weight loss results were dismal. Using biological markers, researchers discovered that most people in the study were eating similar amounts of protein and fat despite the fact they had been assigned different proportions as part of the research design.

All the study participants started out overweight or obese and virtually all ended up that way after two years of intensive coaching and hunger-producing meal plans. The average weight loss was a puny nine pounds. Is this what you want for yourself after two years of struggle?

On the Perfect Formula Diet you can permanently lose nine pounds in one or two hunger-free months. You will eat a satisfying variety of foods. And you can eat all the bananas you want—without measuring them!

Other studies reinforce the findings that, even with dietary counseling, low calorie diets based on reduced portions of typical foods are likely to leave you close to your original weight after a year or two of chronic hunger and feeling deprived, anxious, and guilty.

With diets based on portion control and fewer daily calories, your metabolism slows down so that your Perfect Body adapts to its reduced fuel source. Your digestive system becomes more efficient at absorbing all the calories you do eat.

Exercise alone does not do the trick either. A review of 80 studies showed dietary approaches worked better than exercise alone in getting people to reduce their weight and keep it off. Those who exercised more without changing their eating habits seldom lost more than a minimal number of pounds.

Even an attempt as drastic as bariatric surgery to lose weight and stay trim will only work if you change your eating habits.

Liberation From Weight

You *can* live free from the merciless taskmasters of excess weight, food cravings, and chronic hunger. If you are overweight or obese, your weight is probably a major issue for you just about every day. You worry about what to eat and feel guilty if you have a satisfying meal. You avoid looking in the mirror and grimace when picking out clothes.

Walking, getting into and out of a car, picking something up off the floor, going up a few stairs, and many other daily activities may morph into unpleasant challenges when you are more than your Perfect Weight.

A 2007 survey sponsored by the Calorie Control Council found that 62% of American adults are concerned about dieting all year long. About 29% are dieting at any one time, and each dieter tries an average of four times a year to lose weight, often by cutting down on foods high in sugar, exercising, eating smaller portions, eating foods lower in calories, and skipping meals.

You can be part of the successful group distinguishing itself, losing weight, and keeping it off!

Measuring Your Goals

Body mass index (BMI), a summary of how your weight relates to your height, is the most common measure of whether you are at a desirable weight. Standard practice among researchers is to define a person with a BMI between 25 and 29.9 as overweight, and those with a BMI of 30 or more as obese.

A study of more than 10,000 people in Britain, who were followed by researchers for 13 years, found that those with a BMI between 20 and 22.5 were the least likely to die during the period of the study. Even a BMI in the "healthy" range of 22.5 to 25 gave the person three times the risk of dying from heart disease. Another study of about 41,000 runners found that those with the lowest risk for developing chronic illness had a BMI of less than 22.5.

After reviewing all major cancer studies, a panel of scientists from around the world recommended that people maintain a BMI between 21 and 23 to minimize the chance of developing cancer.

The table later in this chapter shows weights between the BMIs of 20 and 23 that are recommended in these global studies. On the

Perfect Formula Diet, you should find that your Perfect Weight falls into this range and stays there.

Perfect Track Record

People who eat a plant-based diet, with very limited or no animal foods are, on average, significantly thinner than followers of a meat and dairy diet. People also regularly lose weight after adopting a plant-based diet. You will not see these kinds of consistent, impressive findings from ordinary diets.

In the studies that follow, and for the rest of this book, "meat" includes chicken, turkey, and fish as well as "red meat."

- A family practice doctor advised 56 patients to follow a whole-foods diet based almost entirely on plants. The 33 patients who returned for follow up after a year had lost an average of 31 pounds; the 19 who saw the doctor again two years later lost an average of 53 pounds. Patients who followed the diet consistently lost the most weight.
- In a comprehensive review of medical journal articles, 38 out of 40 studies found that those who avoid meat weigh less than people who eat meat even after taking into account differences in exercise. Typically, the meat-free group weighed 6% to 17% less.

  Looking at all the studies as a group, the reviewers concluded that the BMI of those who eat a plant-based diet is lowest. Several studies included in this comprehensive review also discovered that, as the percentage of calories from protein goes up, so does average BMI.
- A study of African-American men revealed that those who ate 100% plants weighed significantly less than those who avoided meat but ate eggs and dairy products.
- Two studies found adults eating mostly plant foods had an average BMI of a healthy and attractive 21, contrasted to a BMI of about 26 for a comparison group of the same age and sex eating a typical American diet. In fact, the plant-based

group had about the same BMI as endurance runners of the same age and sex on a typical American diet.

- In a study of almost 700 men, those who ate a plant-based diet had a significantly lower BMI than either vegetarians (who avoid meat but eat dairy foods and eggs) or meat eaters.
- A study of 25 volunteers on an animal-free diet and 20 matched controls on a typical diet found that those on the animal-free diet had a significantly lower BMI, even though all the volunteers got about the same amount of exercise.
- Researchers compared the weights of 200 California vegetarians, vegans (people whose diet is animal-free), and meat eaters matched for age; those on the animal-free diet weighed, on average, 20 pounds less than their counterparts, even though all the study participants ate about the same number of calories and got about the same amount of exercise.
- Sixty-four overweight and obese women agreed to follow either a 100% plant-based diet with no added oil, or the National Cholesterol Education Program diet (which includes animal foods). The women eating the diet with animal foods cut an average of 388 calories per day from their previous eating habits, while the women in the plant-based group cut 366 calories. In spite of their lesser calorie change, the women on the all-plant diet lost an average of 12.8 pounds in 14 weeks, while the women on a modified "typical" diet lost only 8.4 pounds.
- A group of 19 severely obese Native Hawaiians with an average BMI of 39.6 followed a diet based on unlimited amounts of traditional Hawaiian plant foods, such as taro, sweet potatoes, breadfruit, greens, and fruit for 21 days. During this time, the participants were allowed to eat only tiny amounts of animal foods. In three weeks, the dieters lost an average of 6.4 percent of their weight without being hungry.
- Many Seventh Day Adventists avoid animal foods for religious and ethical reasons. Results of a major study indicate that

Adventists who avoid meat weigh, on average, 13 pounds less than meat-eating Adventists of the same height, even though they all eat about the same number of calories daily. During a 16-year study follow up, those who ate meat were substantially more prone to creep from normal weight to overweight. And animal-free Adventists were, on average, thinner than Adventists eating dairy foods and eggs.

- Another Seventh Day Adventist study found those on an animal-free diet had an average BMI of a healthy 23.6, while those who regularly ate animal foods labored with a BMI of 28.8—well into the overweight range.
- A national survey of more than 10,000 Americans found that those who avoid meat had, on average, a significantly lower BMI than did those who ate meat, despite consuming a higher total quantity of food.
- A study of about 41,000 runners found that those who ate the most meat and fish tended to be the heaviest.

Some of the compelling research focuses on patients with specific health diagnoses.

- Eighteen fibromyalgia patients treated with a diet of raw plant food lost significant weight, compared with 15 patients who continued a diet containing animal foods. Relieving symptoms was the goal of the study; the weight loss in the plant food group was just a nice side effect.
- In a group of almost 900 patients treated for cardiac disease with a diet based mainly on whole plant foods, men lost an average of 12 pounds and women an average of nine pounds over a three month time period.
- Twenty-nine patients with high blood pressure were given instructions to eat a totally plant-based diet for a year as part of a research study; at the end of that time, they had lost an average of 18 pounds.

- Half of a group of 99 adults with type 2 diabetes ate a plant-based diet for 22 weeks. During this time, the other half followed the American Diabetes Association diet. The plant-based diet group lost more—almost 16 pounds in 12 weeks—despite the fact that the two groups rated their diets as equally acceptable and ate about the same number of calories. Those on the plant-based diet did not have to limit portion sizes artificially.

The consistent results keep rolling in from Europe.

- An English study of more than 5,000 adults found that those who did not eat meat were substantially less likely to be obese, and this difference persisted over time, despite the fact that those who avoided meat ate about the same number of calories each day as the meat eaters.
- A study of 183 Dutch men found that those on a macrobiotic diet, which is based on whole plant foods, had the lowest BMI, while those who ate meat had the highest BMI.
- Researchers studying 21 Finnish adults found that those who ate only plants had a significantly lower BMI than similar meat eaters. Yet both groups ate about the same number of calories daily.
- Of 55,000 women in a weight study in Sweden, those who were on an animal-free diet were significantly thinner than the rest of the group.
- An English research project compared 26 people on a 100% plant diet with a group of meat eaters chosen to be as comparable as possible. The plant-based diet group weighed less.
- A European study of almost 38,000 adults found that, for both men and women, those who ate meat had, on average, the highest BMI. Those on a 100% plant-based diet had the lowest BMI. People eating eggs, dairy, or fish, but not meat, were in the middle of the BMI range between the meat eaters and those on the animal-free diet.

Among those who ate any animal foods in this study, the ones who consistently ate the most protein and the least fiber tended to be the heaviest. This finding suggested to the researchers that animal protein is responsible for increasing weight.

Will You Like This Diet As Much As People In The Studies?

Of course, weight loss is not your only consideration in choosing what to eat. Participants in research studies generally liked their plant-based diets, did not feel deprived, and ate when hungry.

The team studying 59 overweight women, assigned either an animal-free diet with no added oil or a "low-fat" diet based on prescribed amounts of typical American foods, asked the women several questions about the eating plans. The animal-free group did not feel any more limited by their study diet than they did in their usual eating pattern, but those on the diet with small amounts of meat did feel more constrained. Both groups felt their assigned diet was equally acceptable in terms of being easy to follow and enjoyable to eat.

Eighty-six percent of those in the animal-free group said they would voluntarily continue their study diet, at least part of the time, after the research was over, and 89% had gotten used to this diet, which helped relieve existing medical problems and was easy to understand without portion control.

Similarly, 99 diabetics in another study were asked to follow either an animal-free diet with no added oil or the American Diabetes Association diet. After 74 weeks, researchers found those assigned to the plant-based diet liked their new eating plan as much as those eating a diet with animal foods.

Researchers found that young women stayed with a meat-free diet, on average, at least two years, but gave up on a calorie-restricted diet after only four months. Another study of 31 overweight women found that 61% voluntarily remained on a near animal-free diet two years after the end of the study they were part of.

You Can Enjoy More Food

Many of the studies described above found that those on a plant-based diet ate at least as much food, and often just as many calories, as those who ate animal foods. You may find it puzzling that studies discover, with such remarkable consistency, that people on animal-free diets are thinner and seldom obese.

One reason for these findings, as you may have guessed, is that the fiber in plant foods is filling and satisfying. Because fiber adds bulk, but cannot be digested by people, foods high in fiber generally have fewer calories per forkful than foods with little or no fiber, such as animal foods or heavily processed plants.

You may be familiar with the idea of energy or caloric density of foods. This simply describes how many calories are in a forkful or plateful of something you might eat. If you stick to foods with lower energy density, you can eat more mouthfuls for the same number of calories, which definitely aids weight loss.

People who avoid meat also tend to have a higher metabolic rate when they're resting than those consuming meat. In other words, even when not exercising, those on meat-free diets are likely to burn more calories each day to produce body heat.

Yet energy density and higher metabolic rates are far from the whole story. Other factors come into play in keeping those on a plant-based diet thinner, including higher insulin sensitivity, healthier levels of growth factors and hormones, and lower levels of systemic inflammation. The rest of this book will help you understand all the reasons a plant-based diet promotes permanent weight loss.

Aim For A Soft Landing

One of the best features of the Perfect Formula Diet is the pace at which you'll move toward your Perfect Weight. You'll aim to lose pounds fast enough to stay motivated as you notice happy changes in your appearance and the way your clothes fit. Yet you don't want to crash your weight too quickly and rebound to your original weight, or even more. Your goal should be a long-term, sustainable coast down to your Perfect Weight.

On the Perfect Formula Diet you'll find you lose a sustainable pound or two a week and never regain it. An excellent reason to strive for this pace of weight loss is the level of toxic chemicals that modern humans have stored in body fat. More than 85,000 industrial chemicals are used in the U.S., with more than 2,000 new chemicals added every year.

Americans of all ages have an average of 116 man-made chemicals in their bodies that should not naturally be present, including DDT, lead, mercury, dioxins, and PCBs. A study of 35 Americans in seven states found that every person had at least seven toxic chemicals (of the 20 tested for) in his or her body—and some had considerably more. Studies described in later chapters link these chemicals to birth defects, cancer, heart disease, asthma, learning disabilities, and other poor health outcomes.

Most of these toxic substances are stored in your body fat. Losing weight too quickly can overwhelm your liver, which is charged with most of the work of getting rid of these harmful substances as they are released during weight loss.

The desirable long-term outcome is that, as you lose weight, your body's load of toxins diminishes, while your health and energy soar. But burning up fat too quickly can lead to feeling ill, as your liver works overtime in the race to detoxify the chemicals that fat cells are releasing.

The Perfect Formula Diet keeps the pace of weight loss to a manageable level. Plus the high amount of beneficial plant nutrients in your meals will help the detoxification process and assist in limiting the damage to your body from the chemicals that are dissolving. Unfortunately, you may feel sick in the initial stages of the detoxification process, no matter what diet you're on.

By basing your diet on whole plant foods in balanced proportions, the Perfect Formula Diet coasts you to your Perfect Weight with welcome health changes and a manageable pace of weight loss as a bonus. You will probably eat a wider variety of satisfying foods than you eat now, without hunger, cravings, arbitrary portion control, or sense of deprivation.

OPTIMAL BMI RANGE-GO FOR IT!

Your Height	Weight (In Pounds) for a BMI of 20	Weight (In Pounds) for a BMI of 23
4'10"	96	110
4'11"	99	114
5'	102	118
5'1"	106	122
5'2"	109	126
5'3"	113	130
5'4"	116	134
5'5"	120	138
5'6"	124	142
5'7"	127	146
5'8"	131	151
5'9"	135	155
5'10"	139	160
5'11"	143	165
6'	147	169
6'1"	151	174
6'2"	155	179
6'3"	160	184
6'4"	164	189

The Story Condensed

Scientists have proven run-of-the-mill diets based on portion control and "lean protein" don't work—though this is not what they wanted to find. Instead, an astonishing perfect track record from around the world shows people on plant-based diets weigh significantly less than those who eat meat, including poultry and fish. Food choice is the key to weight loss, with exercise a distant second.

The BMI range of 20 to 23 is generally ideal for health and appearance. On the Perfect Formula Diet you should coast to this BMI range at a pace that is more manageable for detoxification of manmade chemicals dissolved in your fat than super-fast weight loss would be.

Diet study participants liked plant-based diets—no wonder, since they could eat so much more tasty, satisfying food and still lose weight.

CHAPTER 3

Perfect Foods

Grocery stores offer you three kinds of foods: manufactured foods, animal foods, and Perfect Foods. If you weigh more than you'd like to, one main reason is that you're eating too much of the wrong kind of foods. Just about every diet book will give you this unwelcome message. What you might not realize is that, if you have some extra pounds, *you are not eating enough of the right kinds of food—Perfect Foods.*

It doesn't much matter if you are a fussy eater or have multiple food allergies. There are hundreds of varieties of Perfect Foods, so you are sure to find a rainbow of choices you enjoy.

You will taste the earth, rain, and sun in Perfect Foods. You will reconnect to your roots in the land by choosing nature's true gifts.

You will also be joining the new food evolution, as documented in a study of more than 5,000 consumers. More and more people are adding seasonal vegetables, nuts, berries, organic foods, and whole grains to their eating plans.

Understand Your Cravings: Your Body Is On Your Side
We like to think of our high-tech gadgets as precision machines, but your body must meet standards more exacting than any machine or

electronic device. If your body is to keep on breathing, metaboliz-ing, and sensing, every chemical and physical part of its intricate functioning has to stay in a tight range.

The complexity of your body is unrivaled. Think of all your organ systems—for digesting, breathing, pumping blood, destroy-ing dangerous microbes and chemicals, seeing, hearing, feeling, thinking, reproducing, and more. Each organ system has multiple parts, and all the functions need to work together and with the outside world to ensure your health and survival.

In addition to internal coordination, your life depends on food, water, and oxygen from the environment. To maintain opti-mal functioning, your body has multiple sophisticated inventory control systems to direct you to secure what you need from your surroundings when you're lacking, and to guard against getting so much that the input is toxic.

You want the level of everything you can measure about your body to be right on target—blood pressure, heart rate, temperature, blood sugar, salt, acidity, oxygen, hormone levels, and so on. Your body has numerous complex mechanisms to keep these measures safe and stable, and to stay in the optimal ranges, as long as you get what you need in safe amounts.

Remember, the bulls-eye is in the center of the circle, not above it (too much) or below it (too little).

For food, your body monitors whether you're getting enough calories and nutrients of many types. Receptors in the nerves that line your digestive tract tell your brain what foods are moving through your system and how many nutrients and calories the food contains. In addition, stretch receptors in your stomach tell you how close your stomach is to being empty or topped off. If you're not getting what you need, your body sends you out to get more.

When your inventory control systems tell you to "get more," your ability to refrain from eating is limited. You can resist for a while, and distract yourself from hunger and food cravings, but eventually, you must satisfy the direction of your body and eat. Think of this as similar to holding your breath. You can consciously hold your breath for a short time if you want to. But, sooner rather than later, you have to start breathing again. The urge to breathe is irresistible.

Sure, you can avoid eating longer than you can hold your breath. But eventually, the systems that control your survival are going to triumph and you're predestined to give in to your food cravings.

You may be wondering, if you're getting enough calories, why you would have food cravings. The answer is that the animal foods and manufactured foods you are eating lack essential nutrients your body needs. Calories are not everything. Your body is sending you out to get critical building blocks for health. This is a good thing.

The problem is, because of habit, advertising, convenience, addictive processes, and misinformation about food fostered by big business and industry-friendly bureaucracies, your choices of what to eat don't satisfy your body's needs. Your inventory control systems don't give up—they can't!

Instead, your cravings to eat intensify in an unsuccessful attempt to get what you really need. Although you may crave manufactured foods or animal foods, these choices don't make up for the nutritional lack that is one of the main reasons for your drive to eat too many calories.

Foods That Don't Satisfy

Manufactured foods are usually made in factories and are degraded or stripped down versions of plant foods that started out perfectly healthy. Here are some examples of manufactured foods:

- White flour, white rice, and other refined grains that are the remnants of whole grains.
- Isolated protein powders, from which all parts of food except protein have been stripped, representing protein in a form way more concentrated than the human body was designed to handle.
- Vegetable oils, in the form of oils in a jar or margarine in a tub or a stick. In these isolated, refined oils, all parts of the

food except the fat have been discarded, and the leftovers represent fat in a form definitely more concentrated than the human body is set up for. Liquid and solid vegetable oils tend to be excessively high in pro-inflammatory omega-6 fatty acids.

- Transfats or hydrogenated vegetable oils which have been further chemically altered and, according to scientific consensus, are disastrous for your health. Evidence indicates that transfats promote both heart disease and cancer.
- White sugar, which is a bleached and processed version of naturally sweet plant juices and which, again, is a factory concentrate of parts of a whole plant.
- Artificial sweeteners, chemicals that may fool your taste buds into thinking you're eating something made with sugar, but which don't fool your brain or stomach. You may also try to deceive your body with other artificial food additives, colorings, flavorings, and preservatives. The operative word here is "artificial."
- Foods and drinks made mostly from these refined, artificial, and/or processed components. For example, soda, energy drinks, white bread, many commercial cereals, crackers, cookies, donuts, pies, white pasta, chips, candy, deep fried foods, and many "mock meats" are also manufactured foods.

Genetically modified foods are another type of manufactured food. In this case, the seed is what is manufactured, by mixing the genes of different species in a lab. The resulting plant may look "normal," but at a cellular level is anything but. Does this bizarre genetic mixture of plants and animals sound like a substance that your Perfect Body is designed to thrive on?

Animal foods are the muscles and organs of animals like cows, pigs, lambs, chickens, turkeys, and fish. Animal foods also include the secretions of animals, such as milk and other dairy products from nonhuman mammals, and the reproductive materials of animals—bird and fish eggs.

Neither manufactured foods nor animal foods will top off your nutritional needs, end your food cravings, restore your health, or fuel long-term sustainable and healthy weight loss. In later chapters you'll read about studies that detail some of the harmful effects of eating these types of foods, which you may grow to crave through a process similar to addiction.

Perfect Foods: Permanent Weight Loss And Satisfaction

Think about the characteristics that make a food perfect. If you could have all your wishes satisfied, you might want a food that tastes great, promotes your ideal weight, reduces food cravings, fosters optimum health, keeps you feeling youthful and energetic, and envelopes you in a wonderful aroma. Your food would be visually appealing, convenient, nutritious, satisfying, easy and fun to cook, and inexpensive. You would want the food your Perfect Body is designed to consume.

A truly perfect food would also satisfy your ethical standards for kindness and compassion, promote a green and healthy planet, and move us in the direction of a bright and sustainable future for all.

You might expect that any food with all these characteristics is hard to find because a team of engineers would have to spend years inventing it and working out the manufacturing process. In fact, there are hundreds, even thousands, of Perfect Foods readily and inexpensively available in your local supermarket.

All whole (unprocessed), edible plant foods are Perfect Foods, and have the attributes you want.

Consider the appealing variety of Perfect Foods, grouped into six types.

1) *Vegetables*: lettuce, cucumbers, tomatoes, celery, carrots, bell peppers, radishes, string beans, asparagus, onions, mushrooms,

sugar snaps, snow peas, beets, spinach, kale, chard, collard greens, broccoli, cauliflower, cabbage, brussel sprouts, zucchini, yellow squash, winter squash, turnips, eggplant, okra

2) *Fruits*: apples, bananas, oranges, tangerines, grapefruit, berries, cherries, melons, pineapple, mangoes, plums, peaches, nectarines, apricots, pears, grapes, kiwis, persimmons, pomegranates, lemons, limes, figs, dates, raisins, prunes, avocados, olives

3) *Legumes (beans and peas) and potatoes*: red and green lentils, fresh or frozen peas, dried split peas, and any type of canned, frozen, dried, or fresh beans (black beans, kidney beans, pinto beans, garbanzo beans, white beans, lima beans, fava beans, black eyed peas, soy beans, etc.), and food made wholesomely from beans (including hummus, bean dips, refried beans, soy milk, soy yogurt, miso, tofu, and tempeh) and white, red, yellow, and purple potatoes, sweet potatoes, and yams

4) *Whole grains*: oatmeal, corn, brown rice, barley, bulgur wheat and wheat berries, spelt, buckwheat, rye, millet, quinoa, wild rice, and food made healthfully from whole grains (including whole wheat or other whole grain bread, whole grain pasta, and whole grain cereals)

5) *Nuts and seeds*: walnuts, almonds, peanuts, cashews, Brazil nuts, pine nuts, macadamias, pistachios, coconut, sunflower seeds, sesame seeds, poppy seeds, flax seeds, and other nuts, seeds, and nut and seed butters

6) *Herbs and spices*: garlic, ginger, black pepper, mustard seed, hot peppers, wasabi, fennel, oregano, basil, rosemary, sage, dill, mint, turmeric, chives, parsley, cilantro, nutmeg, allspice, cinnamon, cloves, paprika, cayenne, chili powder, curry powder, coriander, cumin, lemongrass, saffron, bay leaves, vanilla, and many other magnificent tastes and smells

Over the course of human history, people have used at least 3,000 different species of plants for food.

With so many Perfect Foods, the trick to sure and sustained weight loss is to eat each type of Perfect Food in the ideal proportion relative to the other types. This strategy promotes optimal nutrition, hunger and appetite satisfaction, and minimization of food cravings. Chapters 6 and 7 detail these proportions and why the formula works.

Before going into the specifics of this eating plan, it will be helpful to learn more about Perfect Foods in the next two chapters. The better you understand nutrition and reduce your fears about mythical "deficiencies" if you give up manufactured and animal foods, the more consistently and intelligently you will stick to the Perfect Formula Diet.

After all, why should you shortchange yourself? Why should you settle for second-best foods?

Food: It's Not What It Used To Be

Before the days of cheap manufacturing, modern tools, and reliable refrigeration, people lived mostly on Perfect Foods, and on whatever animal foods they could hunt, raise, or scavenge. Animal foods were expensive in terms of resources needed to obtain them and were not the dietary basis for most cultures.

Animal bodies start to decompose as soon as they die, and without refrigeration there were limited ways to preserve large quantities of meat. Because humans are natural plant eaters, they get sick from eating decomposing meat. In addition, fish deteriorate more rapidly after death than other animals. This is because fish largely lack the connective tissue that makes muscle more resistant to spoilage.

Your early ancestors certainly could not afford to kill domestic animals every day, and wild animals are moving targets and not a reliable source of food. Some meat could be salted or dried, but even these technologies evolved relatively late in human history. Hunting tools were crude and not to be relied on for survival.

Most plant foods can be stored much longer than animal food without refrigeration. Plants don't hide, move, or run away, so people developed reliable knowledge about where to find the plants they needed to eat to survive. The ability to see in color, which most animals lack, allowed people to find and choose ripe fruits, vegetables, and other Perfect Foods.

The natural consequence of the low-tech methods of earlier times, which comprise most of human history, is that people ate mostly Perfect Foods, and the human body developed precisely attuned to these foods. *Your body has not forgotten the foods it was meant to thrive on.*

The Story Condensed

You have a choice—animal foods, manufactured foods, and Perfect Foods. Manufactured foods are made from processed plants, manmade chemicals, and genetically manipulated "mad scientist" creations. Animal foods are body parts, secretions, and reproductive materials.

The six kinds of Perfect Foods—whole (unprocessed) plant foods—are vegetables; fruits; beans and potatoes; whole grains; nuts and seeds; and herbs and spices. Perfect Foods are rich in nature's goodness with an irresistible variety of tastes, aromas, and colors. Enjoy them to the max, along with the swelling numbers of others who are rediscovering their true food roots!

CHAPTER 4

Perfect Protein

Protein is the basis of life for *every* living being—plant, animal, or microbe. You may already understand how critical protein is, but everything else you've heard about this substance is probably incomplete or downright incorrect. Protein is a common nutrient you can find abundantly in any Perfect Food. Here is the real story of protein, how it helps you, and how it can harm and fatten you. Be prepared for some surprises!

The public went crazy over the 1838 discovery of protein. Recent diet gurus have largely ignored more than 170 years of protein-related research. You can benefit from the Perfect Formula Diet's 21st century knowledge for weight loss and health.

Your Protein Is Unique

Except for identical twins, no two people have identical proteins in all their cells. More radical differences in proteins make each species of animal and plant different from the others.

Scientists are still researching how many kinds of proteins you make, but estimates range up to a million. Each fulfills a specific job to keep you functioning. The most abundant protein in your body is collagen, which forms your bone, skin, tendons, and cartilage.

Since unique proteins build each of us, and there are wide differences in proteins among different species of plants and animals, how are you able to put together *exactly* the proteins you need? The simple answer you are about to read is key to understanding weight, disease, and health.

All proteins are linked assemblies of smaller units called "amino acids." Just 20 kinds of aminos acids (also called "aminos") form the proteins of all living things. You can use the proteins from parsley and cilantro, potatoes and rice, beans and bananas, to create your own body cells because you disassemble these plant proteins into their aminos during digestion and put those amino acids together again the way *you* uniquely require.

The same thing happens if you eat animal foods—you *disassemble* the protein from that cow or chicken or cheese into its component aminos, and then *reassemble* the aminos according to your own unique genetic blueprint. However, you will learn the many advantages of using aminos from plants instead of animals to satisfy your nutritional needs.

Building Blocks Of Your Life

So what are amino acids made from? Four basic elements—oxygen, carbon, hydrogen, and *nitrogen*—are building blocks of all aminos. These four critical elements make up about 96% of the human body. Some aminos contain small amounts of other substances, such as sulfur.

Carbohydrates and fats are comprised only of oxygen, carbon, and hydrogen. *Nitrogen*, then, is the distinguishing element of protein. In addition to containing nitrogen, protein molecules are generally hundreds or thousands of times bigger than carbohydrate and fat molecules.

You may have heard that farmed animals convert carbohydrates in plants into proteins. Such a transformation would be physically impossible. Because carbs do not have any nitrogen atoms and proteins do, carbs cannot be "transformed" into protein any more than gold can morph into lead.

Earth's Protein Factories

Although there are 20 aminos that together build all plant and animal life, you can simplify this into two important kinds of aminos: the essential and the nonessential. Scientists disagree somewhat on where to draw the line, which can differ by life stage.

A common consensus is that, for people, there are eight kinds of essential aminos and twelve kinds of nonessential aminos. You don't have to eat the nonessential aminos because your body assembles them as needed. The essential aminos must come from your food.

*Plants and micro-organisms (such as bacteria and yeast) are the **only** natural factories on earth for essential aminos, because so much energy is required to put together all the necessary atoms. The sun supplies enough energy, and plants can directly harvest the sunlight through a process called photosynthesis, which happens primarily in leaves.*

All plants, from trees to weeds, must turn non-life into life. To accomplish this routine miracle, *plants* weave oxygen, nitrogen, carbon, hydrogen, and some trace minerals together into amino acids, the building blocks of proteins and all living things—plant and animal.

Sun's Energy Captured

Plants use energy directly captured from the sun to assemble amino acids from molecules in the air and soil. Biologists do not totally understand how plants accomplish this astonishing task, which is the basis for all life on earth.

Why does nitrogen-based fertilizer fuel plant growth? Because nitrogen is the distinguishing element in amino acids, and lots of nitrogen allows plants to manufacture the aminos needed to flourish. On the other hand, a shortage of nitrogen will stunt plant growth.

Proteins make up about 30% of the total dry weight of typical plant cells. Most common food plants assemble the bulk of amino acids in their leaves, and then distribute these essential building blocks throughout the plant for use and storage. Each plant actively regulates the aminos it manufactures, based on its needs and the resources available to it.

Once a plant makes all the amino acids required, it assembles these building blocks into the proteins necessary for its millions of cells to function. There are as many as 20,000 different kinds of proteins in one plant, each actively controlled to optimize the plant's ability to survive and reproduce.

Animals Are Efficient

Animals get 100% of their essential amino acids from plants or bacteria, either directly by eating plants, by eating other animals who consumed plant foods, or from bacteria that live in their gut and make aminos the animal can absorb. Think about that for a minute.

Animals lack the ability to make essential amino acids because they don't have to. These basics of life are readily available through plants. For animals, there is a survival advantage in relying on the environment for abundant resources, rather than having to make them from scratch. Calorie for calorie, green veggies—such as romaine lettuce, broccoli, and kale—have twice as much protein as steak.

You can target plant sources to get your essential aminos and skip the animal middleman. When you eat string beans, apples, rice, peas, oatmeal, or any Perfect Food, your body will use the essential amino acids you digest to build its own cells and tissues.

No matter how much meat you eat, you manufacture your cells 100% from plant-formed or bacteria-formed amino acids. Animal protein is recycled plant protein.

You Link Aminos Into Proteins

Did you ever make a paper chain when you were a child? Think of heavy construction paper cut with blunt children's scissors into thin ribbons of color, ready to be glued into a circle. Remember how you linked each strip to its neighbor before pasting the ends together so you ended up with a long chain for imaginative play?

Your paper chain is an excellent model for understanding how your body makes proteins from aminos. Imagine that the essential aminos are green strips of paper and the nonessential are blue strips. The shades of color are important. There are eight shades of green strips and twelve shades of blue strips. Millions of times each day, your body picks up precisely the strip it needs and joins it to the next strip in the chain. Hundreds or even thousands of amino acid strips form one protein molecule.

To work properly, the amino strips must follow a specific color-coded order, and after the long chain is done, it must be folded or shaped in a precise form to be able to do its job in your body. If even one link in a chain of thousands of aminos is wrong, the entire protein can't do its job right, and you may get sick or even die.

If the chain is a perfect assembly but the folding is faulty, the results can be similarly dire. Mad cow disease and other dangerous disorders are the results of proteins folded incorrectly.

Every cell in your body, guided by your genetics, has the amazing ability to assemble exactly the proteins it needs from amino acids.

Your Body's Closet Space Is Limited

Your body stores extra calories as fat because your ancestors may have survived famine with this back-up. But since amino acids are so abundant in just about any diet, including 100% plant-based eating, your body has limited the amount of aminos you can tuck away for later use. After all, why waste energy and space storing something that won't be needed?

Your body is anticipating a potential calorie shortage, but not a potential amino acid shortage. Your ancestors who stored more amino acids didn't survive any longer than those who did not; otherwise, any flab around your middle would hold protein instead of fat. The amount of protein your body stores is largely dependent on your height and cannot be increased by reasonable food choices.

To better understand your body's design, think of how limited your ability to store oxygen is; only a few minutes without air, and you may die. Why is this? Because oxygen is so abundant in the atmosphere, your body anticipates you will be somewhere you're able to breathe and storing oxygen isn't necessary.

Seals, as an instructive contrast, must spend long stretches underwater to find their fishy foods. Seals are mammals who get their oxygen from the air, the same as humans. Yet the deepest diving seals can stay underwater for one to two hours, which certainly gives them a survival advantage in securing enough to eat. Seals *can* store oxygen, far more than land-dwelling humans, in their enormous blood volume, muscles, special abdominal spaces, and spleen.

The takeaway lesson from the seals is that your body will not waste its resources storing even the most essential basics of life, as long as those necessities are readily obtained in the normal environment. *For humans, protein is as abundant in whole plant foods as oxygen is in the air.*

The Original Recycling

Your Perfect Body has another compelling reason to avoid storing certain amino acids. Some of these building blocks are a toxic threat. Your body specifically targets maintaining these at low levels in its amino acid pools. These deadly aminos must be quickly converted to carbs or fat when you eat too much protein.

While your body's closet space for amino acids is limited, it's not nonexistent. Your body stores some amino acids in higher amounts than others, so the need for specific aminos in your diet is not directly proportional to the composition of protein in your body.

You do lose a tiny bit of aminos every day when skin and intestinal cells die and are not retained by your body. These lost aminos are replaced when you eat; plant proteins fill this role admirably. How about when other cells die?

Luckily, your Perfect Body is an amazingly efficient recycler. If you're an adult, you're probably not growing (larger fat cells don't count here). If you are to form vigorous new cells, old, worn out, or damaged cells need to die. On average, your cells divide 25 million times each second to renew your body.

What happens to the old cells? Your body disassembles them and reuses their constituent parts (including amino acids) again and again and again. Small storage pools of aminos are sufficient to accommodate this recycling. Your body craves energy, not more amino acids, to build new cells.

Remember, an amino acid is a building block. Your body can use it again and again, since it retains its integrity. The amount of aminos lost in this process is tiny. Your body, no matter what your age, is especially skilled at conserving and reusing the essential aminos that are more likely to be in relatively limited supply in your diet.

In 2004, three scientists won the Nobel Prize in chemistry for clarifying how cells break down proteins that are damaged or no longer needed. Each cell has an intricate inventory control system that speedily removes and recycles the targeted proteins. In fact, if this process doesn't happen as it should, then diseases may result. The breakdown of old proteins into their amino acid building blocks is just the other side of the formation of new proteins from the now available components.

Interesting fact: birds generally have higher maintenance amino acid requirements than mammals. Birds use the aminos to grow new feathers as the old ones fall off and must be replaced (the bird cannot recycle the aminos in a feather that has drifted to the ground). Many birds are plant eaters and comfortably meet their high amino acid requirements without animal foods.

Protein: Ideal Amount, Ideal Source

Protein is the most revered nutrient in the mythology of American eating. The popular notion about protein is that more is always better. But too much protein (essentially, too many amino acids) is no better than too much sugar or salt. Remember, you are aiming for the bull's eye, not the top of the outer circle.

According to the World Health Organization, adults need to obtain only 5% of their calories from protein to be healthy. Early studies of protein metabolism showing a higher requirement were performed on rats, who have different nutritional needs than humans.

Human protein requirements are highest in infancy, and the need for protein as a percentage of calories goes down dramatically as people go through childhood and adolescence into adulthood. As an infant grows, his or her rate of making new proteins decreases, regardless of the amount of amino acids eaten.

Human breast milk, the truly Perfect Food for infants, is only 5% to 8% protein, with most calories coming from carbohydrates. The immature organs of infants can be stressed by too much protein. If a food containing no more than 8% protein makes a growing infant flourish, wouldn't less than 8% of calories from protein be more than sufficient for a full grown adult?

Older children, weaned off breast milk, can grow and thrive on an all-plant diet. Children can efficiently use the proteins in rice and corn. As a matter of fact, kids use the protein in potatoes more efficiently than they use casein, one of the proteins in cows' milk. A study of 11 children recovering from malnutrition found that potatoes supplied all the amino acids these deprived children needed to get healthy, as long as the kids got enough calories.

Plant proteins work as well as animal proteins in fueling children's growth to their maximum genetic potential, as long as enough food is eaten. Stunted growth in children is usually related to an undersupply of calories, a monotonous diet, poor public health conditions, and high rates of childhood diseases. While animal protein can promote overly rapid growth, plant protein fuels optimal steady growth resulting in maximum adult height.

Are You Drowning In Too Much Protein?

The amount of protein you need as an adult is slippery to pinpoint, and for good reason. The quantity of protein your body breaks down is, in the short term, determined by the quantity of protein you've been eating for the past several weeks. So protein needs are a moving target and your most recent food choices determine where that target moves.

When you eat too much protein, your body adapts its metabolism to get rid of the excess. "Too much protein" is defined as any amount of protein that supplies more amino acids than your body needs to replace the tiny amount lost each day from normal metabolic processes.

If you stop eating too much protein, your body will keep disposing of the same amount of protein you used to eat before, but only for a short time. Within about two weeks, you'll regain any protein you've destroyed and be back in balance.

This adaptive mechanism accounts for the fact scientists have found that some humans have higher protein requirements. Their subjects are people who habitually eat too much protein and their Perfect Bodies have adapted in order to be able to survive. But these same Perfect Bodies will happily adapt back to a lower protein, less toxic diet in short order.

Who Said More Was Better?

When you eat animal foods, your body gets way more aminos than it needs. Since there's little internal storage space for excess aminos, you have to break down and get rid of the aminos you can't use or store. The by-products of this disposal process are harmful to you.

Your body converts unneeded amino acids into either carbohydrate or fat molecules, which you then burn as fuel or sock away as fat. In fact, if you don't eat enough carbohydrates, your body is forced to turn proteins into sugars and burn them for energy. This happens because key cells in your brain, muscles, and red blood cells must rely almost totally on glucose, one kind of sugar, for all their energy.

To accomplish this conversion of excess amino acids to fat or carbohydrate, you need to eliminate the nitrogen that is in the aminos, but not in the carbohydrate or fat end products. This difficult and complex task stresses your liver, which serves as your excess protein clearinghouse.

On a typical American diet, about half the oxygen your liver uses each day is for converting unneeded amino acids into glucose.

As amino acids are disassembled, poisonous ammonia made from unneeded nitrogen floods your liver. To protect your body, the ammonia is quick changed into a substance called urea as well as other waste products—uric acid and creatinine. People in liver failure may not be able to get rid of protein disposal waste products and go into a coma because of the accumulation of these hazardous substances.

Your kidneys, in turn, need to eliminate the toxic nitrogen-containing waste products of this metabolic process. Not surprisingly, urea and the other leftover substances are excreted in your urine. Eating too much protein (too many aminos) makes your kidneys suffer the wear and tear of filtering your blood faster, one reason that people with kidney disease are usually instructed to eat less protein.

The toxic byproducts of disposing of unneeded amino acids can, therefore, harm your liver and kidneys directly. In addition, animal proteins—which are higher in acidic sulfur than plant proteins—can increase your risk of developing painful kidney stones and osteoporosis. Sulfur from these animal-sourced aminos may also damage the tissues of your intestines and colon.

When your diet has a smaller, optimal amount of aminos, your liver fine tunes how it functions. Enzymes that use the aminos to build protein then dominate your liver's functioning. Aminos are most efficiently recycled and few are converted to carbs or fats.

So if you've been told that sugar is "bad" and you can avoid it by eating "protein," now you know the real story. Your body runs on glucose and will simply transform your animal food into the carbs it needs, unfortunately releasing destructive nitrogen-containing by-products during this process.

Even though, calorie for calorie, some vegetables have more protein than meat, you won't get too high a protein dose from eating veggies because the absolute number of calories in veggies is low. Also, plant foods have lower levels of sulfur-containing amino acids than animal foods. Amino acids that contain sulfur may be especially dangerous to your health when you eat more than you require, because these aminos push your body to be too acidic.

Perfect Foods, Perfect Protein

When you eat Perfect Foods, as long as you're getting sufficient calories, your body gets plenty of amino acids. You don't need to mix and match, or specifically "complement" certain plant foods. Numerous studies have shown that *any* single plant that supplies enough calories to meet your energy needs also supplies all your protein needs. You don't need to "work" to get enough protein on a plant-based diet.

This is because most plant foods supply at least 10% of their calories from protein. People on an animal-free diet get, on average, about 11% of their calories from protein; in contrast, those who eat a typical American diet get about 15% to 17% of their calories from protein. Recall that you require only about 5% of your calories from protein.

Researchers studied a group of 200 people living in California that included plant-based eaters, those who avoided meat but ate dairy foods and eggs, and people who ate meat. While those who avoided meat ate less protein on average, all three groups had comparable levels of proteins in their blood.

Protein Digestion: Transforming Your Food

Your digestive system is designed to break down all the proteins you eat into amino acids before you absorb the food in your intestines. This is true for both plant and animal foods. Your body breaks an average protein molecule down into about 500 amino acids during the digestive process.

Here's something you need to know. Allergic and immune system reactions are responses to foreign proteins—that is, any proteins other than your own. Theoretically, you would never have any proteins enter your body through your digestive tract—only fats, carbohydrates, and amino acids would be absorbed.

If that were the case, food could not provoke your allergic or immune systems. Since people have food allergies, though, some intact foreign proteins, or at least large fragments of the proteins in the form of long amino acid chains, do make it through digestion.

The protein digestive process is about 99% complete. For most people, fragments of intact or partially intact proteins, with the amino acids still linked together, do leak into the blood in small amounts through the intestinal walls. If you were to be tested within hours after a meal, chances are your blood would have antibodies to the animal proteins and maybe even some of the plant proteins that you recently ate.

The reason some intact proteins leak in during digestion is that your intestinal tract has such a delicate job to do. While it must keep out harmful microbes and toxins, it must also absorb essential nutrients. In maintaining this fine balance, some foreign proteins are sure to get through the walls of your intestines. If the walls were so impermeable as to keep out 100% of proteins, then many essential nutrients might also be missed.

Keep Out Those Leaking Proteins

This "leaky gut," as it is informally called, is more severe in people who have inflamed intestinal walls from infection, colitis, inflammatory bowel disease, and allergic conditions. Stress, as well as certain drugs, such as antibiotics, aspirin and NSAIDs (nonsteroidal anti-inflammatory drugs, like ibuprofen), may also make your digestive system more "leaky" to large molecules of intact proteins.

Scientists have also confirmed that, for patients with chronic heart failure, the intestinal barrier is "leaky" and covered with bacteria. The same dangerous state of affairs may underlie cachexia, the distressing body wasting that accompanies cancer and several chronic illnesses.

In Chapters 12 through 15, you'll learn more about how proteins that are foreign to your body can result in system-wide chronic inflammation and a plethora of dangerous, painful diseases. Proteins other than your own can put you at risk for osteoporosis, kidney stones, other kidney disease, high cholesterol, and cancer. In fact, animal protein can directly raise the amount of cholesterol in your blood, in addition to the role that animal fat also plays in this process.

Has Your Old Thinking Gotten You The Results You Want?

You still may be thinking to yourself, "I need animal proteins. Humans have always eaten animal proteins." Difficult as it may be to give up these ingrained ideas, neither is accurate. You don't need animal proteins. Those on a 100% plant-based diet, as a group, thrive compared to people who eat meat. The primates genetically closest to humans are almost exclusively plant eaters.

Compare your fingernails with the claws of a cat. Compare your teeth with those of a true carnivore, such as a cat, rattlesnake, or shark. How could you chase down, kill, and eat an animal or fish without manmade weapons, a campfire, and tools? Would the human body be so poorly designed as to be unable to secure truly essential foods without tools that were invented relatively late in human history?

The enzymes in your saliva are designed to break down complex carbohydrates, which are abundant in Perfect Foods. Animals meant to live on meat have stronger digestive system acids than humans and relatively short and smooth intestines that rapidly rid their bodies of the decaying remnants of their meals. Humans and other natural plant-eaters, in contrast, have long intestines with many small pockets, which give the time and space for plant foods to be completely digested and absorbed.

On factory farms, animals we all know to be plant eaters by nature, such as cows and sheep, are fed meat and are able to digest it. So the fact that humans can digest meat says nothing about our fundamental nature, nutritional needs, or optimal diet.

Humans like the taste of meat only if most of the blood has been drained out of the animal before it's cooked. This is why animals killed for human consumption must have their throats slit while they're still alive, so their beating hearts can pump out most of the blood. Even with the blood drained out, few people like the taste of plain unflavored meat and must disguise it with salt, spices, sauces, smoke, or other seasonings prior to eating it. These flavorings, not the meat itself, evoke the reaction "delicious."

Human taste buds detect and enjoy sweet flavors—your naturally Perfect Body is clearly communicating exactly what it needs. In contrast, cats, true carnivores, have taste buds that detect protein rather than sugar.

A true meat or fish eater, such as a mountain lion, wolf, shark, bear, seal, rattlesnake, or dolphin, bites into its raw, intact prey and consumes the muscles, organs, skin, blood, and bones raw. If this does not appeal to you, or if your teeth and jaws are not equipped to eat a whole raw animal, including skin and bones, then wouldn't it be best to think again about how "essential" animal foods are to you? Once you understand that you have a Perfect Body, the conclusion that you don't require animal protein is undeniable.

Escape The Hype

You may also have read that animal proteins facilitate weight loss. Again, reality is in the opposite direction. Remember vegetarian, factory-farmed animals, such as cows, are fed large amounts of fish meal and other protein-rich animal remains. Why is this done? The reason, since protein promotes rapid growth, is to fatten them up faster so they're ready to be slaughtered at a younger age.

In fact, faster-growing species naturally have higher protein levels in mother's milk. Although human breast milk is only about 5% to 8% protein, rat's milk gets up to 50% of its calories from protein, while cow's milk gets almost 40% of its calories from protein. Quick note: cows naturally eat only plants when not on factory farms, yet have a protein content in their milk that is five to eight times the protein content of human breast milk, even if the human mother lives on animal foods! Nature is wise in regulating how fast a baby will grow, even if the mother makes poor food choices.

Protein can promote runaway growth and weight gain, as later chapters explain in more detail. Several nutrition studies that investigate this issue find that as the percentage of calories from protein in a person's diet rises, so does average BMI.

Think fish will help you lose weight? Go look at a seal. These appealing, torpedo shaped creatures have a thick layer of blubber formed exclusively from the fish and "sea food" they eat. The next time you want to eat fish, form a mental image of a seal, with such a massive layer of fat that she can swim comfortably with icebergs.

Has your old thinking gotten you the results you want in terms of weight, health, and energy level? Are you ready to break free from the protein hype pushed by government bureaucracies and mega-businesses that profit from animal foods?

Since the identical amino acids form plants and animals, why would you have a specific need for "animal protein," which has no secret ingredient missing from plant protein? Why would animal foods be a better source of essential amino acids for you, when the plants manufactured the animals' amino acids in the first place?

You Can Help Kids Who Really Are Malnourished

Kwashiorkor is a disease of protein deficiency in children that occurs when breast-fed infants are weaned too early onto a diet that consists mainly of cassava or green banana. Infants and young children should be weaned onto a varied diet with sufficient amounts of plant foods. Marasmus is a disease that starving children develop when calories are grossly inadequate, with deficient protein resulting from too little total food. True protein deficiency diseases are almost unknown in developed countries.

The best way you can help prevent tragic food deficiency illnesses from decimating young children in poor countries is to eat Perfect Foods. Massive amounts of calories are fed to animals raised for humans to eat. Most of the vitamins, minerals, proteins, and other valuable components in the animal feed are lost and wasted in this process.

If you stop eating meat, the animal feed that is freed up is then available for malnourished people, who otherwise must compete with farmed animals in wealthy countries for food. Do you see how easily you can help nourish hungry children?

The Story Condensed

Every time you see a plant partnering with the sun, you are privileged to witness a miracle in progress as non-life is converted to life. Plants and microbes are the *only* natural factories on earth for putting together essential amino acids, which are the building blocks of all proteins.

There's nothing useful in animal protein that is not also in plant protein; the amino acids used to build the proteins are identical for plants and animals. In fact, animal protein is recycled plant protein.

You don't need a specifically identified "source of protein" in your diet any more than you need a specifically identified "source of oxygen" in your air. Protein is an integral part of all plants in the same way that oxygen is an integral part of the atmosphere.

Unfortunately, animal foods generally have more protein per forkful than plant foods. This over-concentration of protein can lead to health problems as your body struggles to break down and dispose of the excess amino acids. Dangerous by-products and stress on your liver and kidneys are an unavoidable part of this process.

Your digestive system absorbs some food proteins intact rather than disassembled into amino acids. These foreign proteins can provoke your immune system and lead to serious health issues.

Excess protein, usually from animal foods, can fuel runaway growth the same way wood fuels a fire. All living things survive based on controlled growth. Obesity and cancer are two examples of unchecked expansion. You don't want to foster uncontrolled growth in your body any more than you would throw dry branches on an out-of-control fire burning right next to your house.

So when it comes to protein, *more is not better.* Any Perfect Food will supply you with plenty of protein because your body recycles existing amino acids, leaving the net amount you need each day quite small.

CHAPTER 5

Perfect Nutrients

While protein builds most of your body's structure, you need energy to stay warm, move, produce new cells, digest food, fight infections, and breathe. The Perfect Formula Diet includes precisely the right amount and types of clean-burning fuel to keep you lean and vigorous.

And what if you are or aspire to be an athlete? Research shows that athletes do not benefit from a high protein diet or amino acid supplementation. D. Joe Millward, one of the world's foremost experts on human protein needs, calls the amount of additional proteins needed over time by athletes to build lean muscle mass "trivial." Any additional protein that is needed is an integral part of the extra food athletes must eat for the *calories* needed to fuel performance.

Athletes: Perfect Food Fuels Superior Performance
Eating before and during exercise conserves your muscles by preventing your body from breaking down its own tissues for fuel. You must get sufficient *calories* if you're an athlete on an animal-free diet or you may experience a loss in vitality and performance that you mistakenly attribute to lack of animal protein.

Be sure to eat Perfect Food after intensive workouts as well. Your body needs *calories* to refuel and rebuild so you can maintain your energy level and lean muscle. Regardless of the amount of protein you eat, you will lose lean body mass if you do not consume enough total food to supply the calories you need.

Since plant foods generally have fewer calories per plateful than animal foods, you need to eat a larger *volume* of food to get enough calories and maintain the weight your sport may require. Happily, eating is an enjoyable activity, and few will complain about the need to eat more.

Trained athletes don't lose as much protein as newcomers during exercise; the athlete's body adapts over time so there's no net amino acid loss during exercise. If you exercise, you will optimize your body's use of the protein you do eat. As long as you get enough calories, in the long run exercise should not increase your amino acid needs and may even decrease your amino acid needs compared to a couch potato lifestyle.

Studying Athletes Proves The Point

In one study, 12 healthy, normal weight male college students were fed an animal food diet for 20 days. Then the men ate a diet free of all animal foods for 50 days. During that time, 90% to 95% of the protein in their diets came from enriched white flour (a manufactured food stripped of most natural nutrients), with the remainder from small amounts of fruits and vegetables.

During the animal-free period of this study, the men felt they had more energy, and chose to increase their energy expenditure from 3,000 to 3,800 calories a day. At the end of the animal-free period, the men had more lean protein-based body tissue than when that phase started and were in better cardiovascular condition. Think how amazing the results would have been on an optimal plant-based diet!

Another study with healthy students validated the finding that a diet based on wheat protein supplied enough amino acids to fulfill all the requirements of active young adults.

An instructive 1907 study of eight elite Yale athletes had the young men reduce the amount of protein in their diets by 50% over five months by eating all plant foods. During the research period, none of the athletes had decreased strength. In fact, the subjects' strength increased, on average by 35%, and they felt less tired. Some of the athletes had up to an 85% increase in strength on the all-plant diet.

Still another study, comparing a diet based on rice with one that added chicken to the rice, looked at the value of adding animal foods to plant foods to increase the body's protein tissue. Again, researchers chose to work with male students. As long as the men ate an adequate amount of rice, the amount of aminos in their bodies stayed the same or increased. In other words, protein was not an issue on the plant-based diet. *When the men ate chicken along with the rice, the amount of aminos in their bodies did not increase any further.* The researchers concluded that supplementing rice with animal protein had little or no value for the men in their study.

Think about it. If eating animal foods were a sound basis for building muscle and succeeding at sports, athletes could simply eat more animal foods and turn into champions.

These Champs Know How To Eat

Athletes on a plant-based diet take advantage of the edge that Perfect Foods give them in meeting their performance goals. Here are some superfit animal-free athletes who perform impressively.

- Brendan Brazier is an ultra marathon champion and triathlon winner
- Carl Lewis has won 10 Olympic medals in track and field, including nine golds; his best year as an athlete was the year he went animal-free
- Edwin Moses, another Olympic gold medallist, went eight years without losing the 400-meter hurdle competition
- Dave Scott is a six time Ironman world champion
- Tony Gonzales, star football player discovered increased energy and endurance on an all-plant diet

- Dr. Ruth Heidrich, on an animal-free diet for 27 years, is a marathon runner and triathlon winner who has won more than 900 first place medals and ribbons, gaining the honor of being named one of the 10 fittest women in North America at the age of 64 (the other nine women with this elite title were 30 to 40 years younger)
- Seba Johnson, who has never eaten animal foods, is a two time Olympic alpine skier and the first black female alpine ski racer in Olympic history
- Adam Hodges Myerson is a cycling champ
- Scott Jurek is a seven time champion and course record holder for the Western States 100-mile endurance run, defending champion and course record holder for the Badwater Ultramarathon, and *Ultrarunning Magazine* Ultrarunner of the Year for 2003 and 2004, all accomplishments proudly fueled by plant foods only
- Mac Danzig, winning martial arts fighter, observes he can work out longer and recover more quickly on an animal-free diet
- Pat Neshek, skillful Minnesota Twins pitcher, added seven pounds of lean muscle after transitioning to an all-plant diet and different workout program
- Salim Stoudamire is a shooting guard for the Atlanta Hawks
- Other star animal-free athletes include bodybuilders, surfers, wrestlers, tennis stars, dancers, and many other runners and cyclists

Animal Sugar

When you think of animal foods, you probably think of protein, not sugar. In fact, the lactose in milk is a naturally occurring sugar that is partly digested by humans into a sugar called galactose.

If galactose builds up in a woman's body, it can damage her ovaries, increasing her risk of ovarian cancer. For people of both sexes, galactose may damage the inside of blood vessels in the eyes, potentially leading to cataracts. Your adult Perfect Body is not designed to require milk, especially the milk of nonhuman mammals. Many adults are lactose intolerant and have difficulty digesting lactose at all.

The Gift Of 100,000 Nutrients

You may think of eating in terms of protein, carbs, fats, vitamins, and minerals, but there's way more to your food than those few components. Perfect Foods contain health-boosting, nutritionally active compounds called *phytochemicals*, which are not in animal foods and which are diminished in manufactured foods.

Plants make these natural chemicals partly to protect themselves from the strong energy associated with making food from soil, air, and sunshine and from other potential sources of damage. Animals benefit from using these plant-sourced compounds to enhance their own bodies. Science is still in the early stages of identifying these nutrients and determining all the ways they help you.

Phytochemicals include the substances that determine the appealing colors, delightful aromas, and delicious flavors of Perfect Foods. While your body may not have a need for a specific amount of each kind of phytochemical, these substances, when eaten in Perfect Foods, help guard your body against injury and disease at the cellular level.

Studies indicate there may be up to 100,000 different kinds of phytochemicals. Researchers and dietitians appreciate the importance of phytochemicals in optimizing human health and nutrition. Only a small percentage of the ability of whole plant foods to destroy harmful substances in your body comes from familiar vitamins; most of the beneficial effect comes from phytochemicals.

Good Things Come In Perfect Packages

Phytochemicals are ideally packaged in Perfect Foods in *exactly* the best amounts and proportions for your body. These valuable substances in plants work as part of a superstar team, not in isolation. Examples of phytochemical types are lignans, isoflavones, resveratrol, and flavonoids, each of which contains several subcategories.

The synergistic blend of phytochemicals in Perfect Foods can encourage detoxification, neutralize free radicals and protect your DNA, balance your immune system, guard brain functioning, ensure your genes are expressed in the most favorable way possible, keep hormones at ideal levels, reduce inflammation, prevent blood clots, reduce blood pressure, and attack bacteria and viruses.

Here's a great example. Researchers have found that women who eat more lignans and isoflavones, both of which compete with estrogen in binding to estrogen receptors in people, have a reduced risk of breast cancer. Flavonoids are the substances in dark chocolate and tea, among other foods, pinpointed as most likely to be beneficial for cardiovascular health, cancer prevention, and other health benefits.

An exhaustive study of all the kinds of phytochemicals and the specific health benefits of each would take an entire book, and might not contribute much to your health. For example, there are more than 170 phytochemicals in an orange. You would have a difficult time choosing between the beneficial phytonutrients in broccoli vs. those in oranges. The solution, the Perfect Formula Diet, will envelope your body with so many phytochemicals that you'll feel comfortable never having to choose either/or.

If a little is good, a lot is *not* necessarily better. In fact, too much can be toxic.

Phytochemicals in Perfect Foods cannot be duplicated with store-bought supplements. Such manmade pills isolate only a few phytochemicals, and then deliver those in doses more concentrated than your body is designed to handle.

You cannot get too many phytochemicals from eating Perfect Foods, but you might from eating manufactured versions of bits and pieces of these healthy substances.

Manufactured Oils: How To Turn
A Good Plant Bad

Imagine a Perfect Food, such as corn or sunflower seeds. If eaten whole, this food could fuel health and weight loss. Now visualize this food disassembled in a factory into its components, with virtually all of the food value degraded or lost.

One of the factory products is vegetable oil. You may be used to thinking of such oil as "natural," healthy, even essential. But in fact, separating the oil from the whole plant is a relatively recent process. To be usable in cooking, most vegetable oils need to be heavily refined because otherwise the oils would quickly develop an unpleasant smell and appear quite unappetizing.

In a factory, the oil extracted from the rest of the plant is processed to remove moisture and "impurities," which are the parts of the plant other than the oil. During this process, caustic soda is added to the oil so some of the impurities become an insoluble soap that settles out. The resulting mix is further bleached and deodorized to make the product consumers expect to see. This manufactured substance is then jarred, as the oil will deteriorate rapidly if exposed to air.

Clearly this entire process is a latecomer to human history and is totally dependent on recent technology. In fact, most refined vegetable oils did not find their way into the human diet in any quantity until 1913. So these oils could hardly be essential to your Perfect Body, designed to thrive on foods found in nature.

In addition, when refined vegetable oils are heated, their structure changes even further from their natural form in the plant, and toxic substances may result.

Most manufactured vegetable oils have concentrated levels of omega-6 fatty acids, which can raise the risk of cancer, depression, and other maladies. Chapter 15 outlines in more detail the pro-inflammatory effects of omega-6 fatty acids and the anti-inflammatory effects of omega-3 fatty acids.

Oils Manufactured From Animals

Just as only plants can produce essential amino acids, only plants can produce essential fatty acids. You're likely to be healthiest when you obtain your omega-3s from plants and, again, cut out the animal middleman.

Early in human history, your ancestors ate wild plants, which have more omega-3 fatty acids (relative to omega-6s) than cultivated plants. However, flax seeds have a high concentration of omega-3s and ground flax seed is the most convenient source of omega-3s in modern societies, as well as an excellent source of lignans and other phytochemicals. In addition to flax seeds, green leafy vegetables, soybeans, and walnuts are good sources of omega-3s.

Fish provides you with omega-3s *only* to the extent that the fish ate algae or other wild plants that make omega-3s or ate other fish that ate such wild plants. *Fish cannot, on their own, form omega-3s.* Farmed fish have fewer omega-3s than do wild fish, because they don't live on plants that grow wild in their habitat.

The omega-3 fatty acids in fish tend to be unstable after the fish is dead, producing free radicals that can damage your body. Fish oil will naturally deteriorate even more quickly than vegetable oil. To make fish oil for human consumption, factories must heavily process and refine the fish bodies.

You may have been told that only fish oil supplies "long chain" omega-3 fatty acids, and the "short chain" omega-3s in plants are not as good. But again, the "long chain" acids originate in marine algae, not in fish. You can readily find "long chain" omega-3 supplements based on marine algae, if you are convinced you need a supplement (see Chapter 21, *Perfect Resources*).

How Your Ancestors Thrived

Here's some great news. Your body makes its own "long chain" omega-3s naturally from the "short chain" omega-3s in ground flax seed and other plant foods.

The enzyme needed for this assembly process will not be abundant as long as you eat too many omega-6s relative to omega-3s, or if you eat hydrogenated vegetable oils or meat. This is another great reason to skip the manufactured vegetable oils.

Researchers gave 56 adults with chronic illness "short chain" omega-3 fatty acid. Within 12 weeks, the study participants had higher levels of the desirable "long-chain" omega-3s in their blood. The researchers concluded that "short-chain" omega-3 is effective in boosting the body's level of "long chain" omega-3s, even in people who were not eating a particularly healthy diet.

Remember, no matter how much fish or fish oil you eat, your omega-3 fats originate entirely in plants. Think about it and the fish oil hype will evaporate for you.

Why Shortchange Yourself?

Manufactured oils are no more nutritious or necessary than refined sugar or white flour—but are a more concentrated calorie source, with about 100 calories in just one tablespoon. When you use oils to prepare foods, buy foods cooked in oil, or eat fat-laden animal foods, it's easy to get 30% to 40% of your calories from fat. If you eat whole plant foods, about 10% of your calories will be from fat. This difference—about 400 to 600 calories from fat each and every day (based on a 2,000 calorie daily diet)—adds up to 40 pounds or more of weight on your body a year.

So if you use a typical amount of manufactured oils and animal fats, you may gain 40 pounds a year from this food alone. Or, to keep your weight steady, you need to cut back on nutrient-dense foods that supply essential elements for health. Either way, you shortchange yourself when you use manufactured oils.

Fooling Your Own Body: Why?

Manufactured food can be overly sweetened, as well as full of refined oils. If you eat manufactured foods with artificial sweeteners, you may be trying to enjoy the appealing taste of sugar without the calories. Bottom line—you are trying to fool your taste buds and your own body. Once you understand the need to work with your Perfect Body to permanently lose weight, you'll see use of artificial sweeteners can backfire. When it comes to lifelong weight loss, honesty is the best policy.

In one study, researchers gave 24 normal-weight people yogurt an hour before lunch, then measured how much each person ate at lunch and the rest of the day. The yogurt was prepared in one of four ways:

- Unsweetened
- Artificially sweetened
- Sweetened with sugar to taste as sweet as the artificially sweetened yogurt
- Supplemented with added starch

The researchers discovered that those who ate the artificially sweetened yogurt ate the most calories from lunch through bedtime. Those who had the starch-supplemented yogurt ate the least the rest of the day.

In another study, researchers gave 120 people gum with different concentrations of artificial sweetener. This gum led to a short-term decrease in reported hunger in most of those tested, followed by a sustained increase in how hungry the people said they felt.

So while calories suppress appetite, a sweet taste can boost appetite; and a sweet taste without calories may boost appetite the most. Eating intensely over-sweetened food can also dull your taste buds, so a whole food that is naturally just a little sweet can seem bland by comparison.

Remember, your body has complex sensors to tell your brain what was in your food. While artificial sweeteners may fool your tongue, your sensors for calories know what has really just landed in your stomach and will send you out to get more food if they're disappointed. Trying to trick your body into thinking you're full when you're really hungry is pointless and counterproductive.

Minerals Come From Rocks

Minerals, such as calcium, iron, zinc, potassium, and selenium, are naturally found in the rocks and soil of our planet. The roots of plants absorb minerals dissolved in the water in soil, and incorporate these minerals as a necessary part of the plants' structure and metabolism.

Animals eat the plants and obtain the minerals in the soil through the plants' ability to absorb these elements. If the water animals drink (for example, natural stream water in the days when streams and rivers ran pure) contains dissolved minerals, then animals can also get needed minerals from this natural source.

Animals cannot make or manufacture any minerals—including calcium, iron, and zinc. For example, the calcium in cow's milk did *not* originate in the cow. The calcium came from the cow's plant food and water. You can get all your minerals in the same place the cow got hers and be optimally nourished through nature's original design.

Perfect Foods have all the minerals you need, as long as you eat a sufficient variety on the Perfect Formula Diet. *Meat and milk are not the original sources of your calcium or any other minerals. Plants and sometimes drinking water are the genuine originators of all the minerals your body needs.*

The Story Condensed

Because plants are the most efficient and effective source of nutrition, the largest land animals are all plant eaters. Think of elephants, buffalo, gorillas, giraffes, horses, and cows. What does this tell you about the best source of energy, protein, fatty acids, and minerals? Additionally, athletes on an animal-free diet can become more effective and therefore champions.

Only plant foods contain the beneficial, nutritionally active compounds called phytochemicals. Every bite of Perfect Foods fortifies your body with these powerful protectors.

The essential fatty acids and minerals in your body all originate from plants or drinking water. Manufactured plant oils in bottles or tubs are usually skewed in favor of inflammatory omega-6 fatty acids. *Animals do not manufacture either essential fatty acids or minerals, so you don't have to eat animals for these essential nutrients.*

Famine and deprivation have stalked human history. If you have ready access to a wide range of affordable and appealing foods, you're extremely lucky. With knowledge and commitment, you can join the growing community of people making wise choices about what to eat, what to avoid, and how to regain and maintain a Perfect Weight.

Imagine how wonderful you'll feel eating plates and bowls full of tasty, satisfying Perfect Foods. In all the world, there's no treat more delicious or filling than a home-cooked meal of Perfect Foods shared with family and friends.

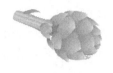

CHAPTER 6

Perfect Formula Diet

If you ever enjoyed a crunchy apple, fluffy baked potato, filling black beans, creamy oatmeal, or a fresh green salad, you're already well on your way on the Perfect Formula Diet. Now you can complete what you started.

When you eat Perfect Foods in ideal proportions, you lose weight and stay lean without hunger or complex food tracking systems. Erase the term "portion size" from your vocabulary. You don't dissect your foods into carbs, fats, and proteins. No need to stress about calcium or iron. Take fiber and the glycemic index off your list of things to fret about. Calories count, but you don't count calories. Your food will come perfectly packaged with the nutrients and energy you require. What could be more convenient?

Just focus on eating enough Perfect Foods to satisfy your hunger using the Perfect Formula Diet. Stop eating when you're no longer hungry. This will be easier for you than it is now because your food cravings will diminish. That's all there is to it.

Remember the story of Goldilocks and the three bears? Well, this is the "just right" eating plan. Forget the high "this" and low "that" diets (high protein, high fat, low fat, low carbs, or whatever is confusing you). The Perfect Formula Diet is effortless balance.

Now you're working *with* your Perfect Body, so you can focus your enhanced energy on projects other than dieting and weight. If you're still stuck in an old habit of concern about deficiencies, then avoid a deficiency of Perfect Foods.

The Perfect Formula Diet builds on the new Four Food Groups— vegetables, fruits, whole grains, and legumes—identified by the extraordinary non-profit Physicians Committee for Responsible Medicine (PCRM). Many other physicians and nutritionists are now realizing the transformative power of a diet based on minimally processed plant foods.

Are you seeing fruit served more often at meetings and as snacks? In many communities, natural food stores are opening or supermarkets are adding special sections of healthier choices. Join the community of people getting back to their true food roots and thriving on this 21st century diet.

Important Note On Medical Conditions And Drugs

The Perfect Formula Diet can enhance your health as well as the appearance of your waistline. Chapters 12 through 15 on health explain how. If you're being treated for a chronic disease with drugs, insulin, or other prescribed treatments, then the additive effects of the Perfect Formula Diet *and* your existing treatment need to be tracked. For example, your blood pressure or your blood sugar level could fall too low (if you are currently taking drugs to lower high blood pressure or insulin or other drugs to control diabetes).

If you have a diagnosed chronic illness or are on medication, it is critical that you work closely with your physician before beginning the Perfect Formula Diet and while you're on this diet, until your body chemistry is stabilized at healthier levels and new doses of drugs or insulin (if these are still necessary at all) are established. In no case should you change the dose of or discontinue any prescription or non-prescription drug, except under the supervision, and with the consent, of an appropriate, licensed health care professional.

If you have a chronic condition, please do not let this precaution deter you from following the Perfect Formula Diet; just do it under your physician's supervision. As your health blossoms and your weight coasts to its optimum, you'll be astonished by how much better you feel and by your minimal need for drugs or other treatments.

The Perfect Formula Diet

A formula is a scientific rule for getting to a specific result. The Perfect Formula Diet is an easy-to-follow method of combining Perfect Foods to lose weight and improve your health. Consistently following the Perfect Formula Diet will put you at your Perfect Weight.

Remember the six categories of Perfect Foods, including:

Vegetables: lettuce, cucumbers, tomatoes, celery, carrots, bell peppers, radishes, string beans, asparagus, onions, mushrooms, sugar snaps, snow peas, beets, spinach, kale, chard, collard greens, broccoli, cauliflower, cabbage, brussel sprouts, zucchini, yellow squash, winter squash, turnips, eggplant, okra, etc.

Fruits: apples, bananas, oranges, tangerines, grapefruit, berries, cherries, melons, pineapple, mangoes, plums, peaches, nectarines, apricots, pears, grapes, kiwis, persimmons, pomegranates, lemons, limes, figs, dates, raisins, prunes, avocadoes, olives, etc.

Legumes (beans and peas) and potatoes: red and green lentils, fresh or frozen peas, dried split peas, and any type of canned, frozen, dried, or fresh beans (black beans, kidney beans, pinto beans, garbanzo beans, white beans, lima beans, fava beans, black eyed peas, soy beans, etc.), and food made wholesomely from beans (including hummus, bean dips, refried beans, soy milk, soy yogurt, miso, tofu, and tempeh) and white, red, yellow, and purple potatoes, sweet potatoes, or yams

Whole grains: oatmeal, corn, brown rice, barley, bulgur wheat and wheat berries, spelt, buckwheat, rye, millet, quinoa, wild rice, and food made healthfully from whole grains (including whole wheat or other whole grain bread, whole grain pasta, and whole grain cereals)

Nuts and seeds: walnuts, almonds, peanuts, cashews, Brazil nuts, pine nuts, macadamias, pistachios, coconut, sunflower seeds, sesame seeds, poppy seeds, flax seeds, etc., and nut and seed butters

Herbs and spices: garlic, ginger, black pepper, mustard seed, hot peppers, wasabi, fennel, oregano, basil, rosemary, sage, dill, mint, turmeric, chives, parsley, cilantro, nutmeg, allspice, cinnamon, cloves, paprika, cayenne, chili powder, curry powder, coriander, cumin, lemongrass, saffron, bay leaves, vanilla, and many other magnificent tastes and smells

The Perfect Formula Diet balances each of these categories of Perfect Foods against the other. By **volume:**

> One quarter of your food will be *vegetables*
> One quarter of your food will be *fruits*
> One quarter of your food will be *legumes (beans and peas) and/or potatoes*
> One quarter of your food will be *whole grains*

You can use whatever measure of volume you like; for example, a half cup or a cup would be convenient.

Picture a merry-go-round with four brightly painted wooden horses equally spaced. Imagine that every time a horse passes you, the rider hands you a plate or bowl of food. One rider gives out vegetables, the next flavorful fruits, the third alternates bean and potato dishes, and the fourth gives you a hunk of whole grain bread, a filling bowl of oatmeal, or another whole grain treat.

To this food rotation, add a handful of *nuts* or a tablespoon or two of nut or seed butters four to six days a week.

In addition, be sure to eat two tablespoons a day of *ground flax seeds*. This will be your reliable source of sufficient omega-3 fatty acids, which will be in healthy balance to your omega-6 fatty acids as long as you don't use manufactured oils.

Remember, the flax seeds must be finely ground so you can digest and use them. A coffee grinder is the ideal tool to grind the seeds, or you can buy them already finely chopped at many grocery stores. Blenders and food processors don't usually do an adequate job of pulverizing the flax seeds.

Eat flavorful foods with generous amounts of fresh or dried herbs and spices. You can make your food spicy with hot peppers or hot sauce if you like; or simply keep the seasoning mild but still tasty and aromatic with herbs and spices that don't burn your tongue. It's your preference; either is fine. These flavorings satisfy your appetite and boost your health by providing a concentrated source of beneficial phytochemicals. Your food will have so much character from these seasonings that you'll want little, if any, added salt.

There are no pre-established "portion sizes" or "servings" with the Perfect Formula Diet. Simply eat when you're hungry and stop eating when you're satisfied.

Aren't you tired of run-of-the-mill diets that warn you to ignore hunger, one of your strongest instincts? What if a diet told you not to breathe—it's not very different. Now you can clearly see how your former diet attempts were doomed to failure. *This time will be different!*

Not-Meal Plans

This book doesn't contain meal plans because eating is not limited to "meals." Tying your eating decisions to the clock can be a recipe for struggle because your Perfect Body operates on its own time and rhythms.

Feel free to "snack" or skip meals altogether and just graze when your body signals that you need food. If you wait until you're extremely hungry, you're more likely to overshoot your body's true nutritional needs and eat too much. You'll be most successful if you eat when you're slightly to moderately hungry.

Here's one idea of how to start the Perfect Formula Diet with an uncomplicated and stress-free strategy. Write down three in-season foods you enjoy in each category of Perfect Foods. For the first day or two you can simply choose to rotate these foods. This is your initial "not-meal" plan that you can expand on whenever you want.

Here's an example. Imagine the following are your favorite foods in each group (of course you will substitute whatever foods are most appealing to you).

> Vegetables—string beans, asparagus, tomatoes
> Fruits—apples, pears, bananas
> Beans/potatoes—black beans, russet potatoes, red potatoes
> Whole grains—oatmeal, whole wheat bread, corn
> Spices—cinnamon, garlic, black pepper
> Nuts—walnuts, peanuts, pistachios

Depending on your appetite and schedule, you could start the day at 7 a.m. with oatmeal mixed with cinnamon, sliced pears, two tablespoons of ground flax seed, and a bit of soymilk. At 9:30 a.m. perhaps eat a peanut butter sandwich on whole wheat bread (okay to use a small amount of jelly on the sandwich).

At 12:30 p.m. eat some boiled red potatoes and a bowl of black beans mixed with chopped tomatoes and garlic. Later in the afternoon eat apples and bananas. At 6 p.m. enjoy corn on the cob, a baked potato with black pepper and roasted garlic, steamed asparagus and string beans. If you are hungry later, eat a couple of walnuts or pistachios and a pear.

The next day you can follow the same plan if you want. By the third day, you will likely be ready to branch out and add more foods and new recipes.

Notice no amounts are specified in this not-meal plan. This is because you are going to eat when you are moderately hungry and stop when you are full.

Do you see how simple this can be? There is no need to stress or cook elaborate recipes unless you want to.

You are probably used to diets that specify meal plans for a month, with "portion control" for virtually every food. The not-meal plans you put together yourself for the Perfect Formula Diet avoid the problems of this routine approach.

The meal plans in traditional diets are likely to leave you unsatisfied. The foods included may be out of season, expensive, or not foods that you like. Worst of all, because you are following someone else's plan, your level of commitment will probably fall off quickly. You will have a much easier time following a plan you put together yourself, precisely because this requires some initial effort on your part.

More Not-Meals To Satisfy Your Taste Buds
Here are more ideas for not-meal plans. Combine the foods you like into your old favorites, modified for Perfect Foods.

For example, you can savor:

- Sandwiches
- Wraps
- Burritos
- Enchiladas
- Tamales
- Pasta dishes
- Rice dishes
- Soups
- Stews

- Salads
- Stuffed baked potatoes
- Chili
- Casseroles
- Stir-fries
- Pizzas

Use your own recipes, the recipes suggested in *Perfect Resources* at the end of this book, or just spur-of-the moment creativity. Whole grain cereal with ground flax seed, cinnamon, dairy-free milk, and sliced fruit is a filling and fast one-bowl delight you can enjoy any time of day or evening.

Vary the themes of your not-meal plans by using a variety of fresh and dried herbs and spices. For example, basil, parsley, and oregano add an Italian flair, while cumin, cilantro, hot sauce, salsa, chilies, and chili powder lend a Mexican touch. Stir-fry in water, vegetable broth, juice, or wine instead of oil.

On the other hand, your thinking has long been guided by breakfast, lunch, and dinner categories. Feel free to eat at mealtime and only mealtime if that works for you. There's no particular food that's better at one meal than at another. You can eat fruit for breakfast, but it's equally good for dinner. The leftover soup or burritos you make from Perfect Foods for a weekend lunch can be any meal on Monday.

The Most Liberating Diet

While the Perfect Formula Diet is undoubtedly a major restructuring of your food habits, transitioning can be comfortable and amazingly painless. The rest of this book shows you how to make that transition and toughens your motivation and commitment.

If you're used to a diet based on manufactured and animal foods, the Perfect Formula Diet will appear unfamiliar. You may worry about feeling deprived and focus on the things you no longer will be eating—animal foods and manufactured foods. *But to feel deprived is a choice; by a simple readjustment of attitude, you can just as easily feel liberated.*

- You *can* still eat anything you want. It's perfectly legal. It's just that you *choose* to eat Perfect Foods. This distinction is critical. If you make a free and conscious decision to change your diet, as so many others have, you can take the attitude that you're simply liberating yourself from old food habits and moving on to something healthier. No one is forcing you to do anything.
- You're liberating yourself from hunger between meals, tiny meals that leave you wanting, complicated diets that force you to count what you eat, diets that make you sick or constipated, diets that result in unpleasant weight fluctuations because they simply don't work in the long run, diets that intensify your food cravings, and diets based on unsustainable foods that harm our planet and threaten our children's future.
- You're liberated from overweight and obesity and the many associated horrific health consequences.
- You're liberated from worrying about, counting, and measuring the individual components of foods, such as proteins, carbs, fats, vitamins, and minerals.
- Depending on your current health, you may enjoy the good fortune of liberation from many hours and significant dollars devoted to health practitioners and drugstores.
- You'll almost certainly be enjoying new foods and a tastier rainbow of foods than you ever ate before.
- You'll be joining the legions of people making exciting new food choices.

Forget what you won't be eating and enjoy the wonderful spectrum of filling and flavorful foods you will be savoring.

*The quality of your life does **not** go down when you stop eating a current food you like. The quality of your life does, however, take a dive when you're overweight, aging quickly, and don't feel your best.*

You'll soon transition to healthier foods you'll grow to enjoy even more than the foods that are making you overweight and sick.

More On The Perfect Formula Team

The Perfect Formula Diet ensures that you're fueled by nature's finest offerings. Your food is dense with nutrients, flavors, colors, and aromas. The variety and combinations of foods are endless.

Here's the best news. Your Perfect Body will finally have both the calories and nutrition it needs to be satisfied and function at its best. Food cravings will diminish, and your enthusiasm for the diet will grow as you feel better, shed pounds, share wonderful new choices with your friends, and find new and interesting foods to keep your taste buds excited.

Expect a gentle glide as you coast to your Perfect Weight. Many people will lose a pound or two a week. This pace of shedding pounds is far easier for your body to handle without ill effects than if you lose weight faster. Any drop in weight will be cumulative and sustained as long as you follow the Perfect Formula Diet.

When you first begin this eating plan, you may lose weight more quickly. This initial faster pace of weight loss is okay. You don't need to worry, as long as you're following the Perfect Formula Diet and eating when you're hungry.

The merry-go-round image of the four horses will help you remember the basics of the Perfect Formula Diet. Another mental picture that may be helpful is a four-cylinder engine. Vegetables, fruits, beans and/or potatoes, and whole grains form the cylinders. Your aim is to fire on all four cylinders on your way to your Perfect Weight and Perfect Health.

Write down or draw a memory aid to help you recall the groups of Perfect Foods in your eating plan. Making the memory aid yourself—whether it is simply a list or a more elaborate visual—will help you understand, remember, and select the foods that make you thrive.

In practice, there is no need to eat the various types of Perfect Foods in any particular order. Aim for a rough balance of the four major categories (vegetables, fruits, beans and/or potatoes, and whole grains) in terms of volume as indicated over the course of a day or two. For example, it's perfectly okay to eat two or three pieces of fruit in a row. Before or after you do this, just make sure to eat enough of the other categories of Perfect Foods.

You don't need to precisely quantify the amount of anything you're going to eat. A rough judgment should be fine for most people. If you want to use a measuring cup or find it helpful, then go for it. But this degree of precision is not required to achieve the results you want. Just be sure you approximately balance the four major kinds of Perfect Foods so you eat these in generous and similar amounts.

Strive to eat a variety of choices within each category of food type. For example, for fruits, eat as many kinds as you can. If you eat only apples and bananas, you'll still benefit, but not as much as if you added six or eight other kinds of fruit to your menu of choices. Each food has its own unique benefits and you want to reap the advantages of as many Perfect Foods as you can. Combinations of many kinds of Perfect Foods work together to maximize your health.

Think of Perfect Foods as your health team. The more strong players, the better you're likely to look and feel. So maximize your health by choosing a large and diverse lineup of whole plant foods.

The Story Condensed

The Perfect Formula Diet balances each category of Perfect Foods against the other. By **volume**:

> One quarter of your food will be *vegetables*
> One quarter of your food will be *fruits*
> One quarter of your food will be *legumes (beans and peas) and/or potatoes*
> One quarter of your food will be *whole grains*

To this food rotation, add a handful of *nuts* or a tablespoon or two of nut butters four to six days a week. In addition, be sure to eat two tablespoons a day of *ground flax seeds*.

Eat flavorful foods with dazzling herbs and spices that you enjoy. The phytochemicals in the herbs and spices help satisfy your appetite and diminish food cravings.

The sooner you start following the Perfect Formula Diet, the quicker you'll get to your Perfect Weight! Why be overweight longer than you have to?

Surprisingly, the truly impressive array of benefits from this eating plan comes from a relatively modest change in lifestyle—modifying food choices. Not everyone is successful at dieting. But if you follow the Perfect Formula Diet, you'll be in the successful group.

CHAPTER 7

Perfect Rotation

Initially, you'll probably enjoy some Perfect Foods more than others and will be tempted to stick to just eating your favorites. But here's what you need to understand. When each category of Perfect Food is balanced against the others, you'll be most successful. Each has a critical role to play in your sustained weight loss and health.

Rotating the Perfect Food categories has significant advantages:

- You'll alternate the foods with the highest amounts of nutrients and lowest number of calories per bite (vegetables and fruits) with foods that have enough calories to turn off your appetite and make you feel full (beans, potatoes, whole grains).
- Rotating provides an endless variety of satisfying, appealing, and delicious foods all year long.
- Some foods are more portable than others for traveling, and others are more commonly available in restaurants or grocery stores when you're not at home.
- You get a wide range of naturally balanced vitamins, minerals, and phytochemicals to foster super health and diminish or end food cravings. Research demonstrates that every food

category forming the Perfect Formula Diet has important health benefits and each has its own nutritional profile.

- You'll get the full range of phytochemicals to help your liver detoxify the chemicals released as your body fat dissolves.
- You can best control the cost of food by buying in season and balancing generally less expensive foods (beans, potatoes, and whole grains) against sometimes more costly foods (fresh fruits and vegetables).
- You include some foods that are probably already a mainstay of your diet with more unfamiliar foods, giving you time to adjust to new flavors and textures.

The Numbers Add Up For You

The Perfect Formula Diet allows you to eat generous amounts of food and still consume few enough calories for weight loss. Here are the calculations. Your stomach can accommodate about one liter of food at a time. Because your stomach generally still has some food in it when you start to eat, you don't need to consume an entire liter of food at a time to feel satisfied.

Perfect Foods have different numbers of calories per liter. These are approximate figures:

- Vegetables: 200 calories per liter
- Fruits: 300 calories per liter
- Beans, peas, and lentils: 500 calories per liter
- Potatoes: 600 calories per liter
- Whole grains: 1,000 calories per liter

So if a liter of food you just ate is one quarter vegetables, one quarter fruits, one quarter of an equal mixture of beans and potatoes, and one quarter whole grains, then you'll have just eaten about 513 calories total.

A liter is a little bigger than a quart. You're not likely to sit down and eat a quart of food at a time. This is especially true if you're eating whole plant foods packed with filling fiber. In fact, if you eat nine cups of food a day, which may be even more than you already eat on your standard diet, you would have just eaten about 1,080 calories of jammed-pack, satisfying nutrition.

If you add 300 calories from nuts and seeds and 100 calories from occasional treats (discussed later in this chapter) as a daily average (the exact number could vary from day to day), you would just have eaten about 1,480 calories on a typical day. This would allow you to feel quite satisfied and still lose a pound or two a week.

The point of these calculations is *not* to tell you to eat nine cups of food or any particular number of calories a day. Your Perfect Body will tell you when and how much to eat through the hunger signals it sends. The point is that you can eat a lot of food and still attain and maintain your Perfect Weight.

Vegetables: No Controversy Here

Have you ever met a reputable person who claimed that vegetables aren't healthy and not an integral part of healthy weight maintenance? Okay, so here's one part of your diet that won't be in dispute.

You probably already have a goal to eat more vegetables. The Perfect Formula Diet helps you meet that objective by combining low calorie veggies with higher energy Perfect Foods of other types.

Your best practice is to make dark green leafy vegetables at least one of your rotations of this whole food group each day. The color indicates a high concentration of chlorophyll, the potent green substance responsible for transforming solar energy into biological energy. Leaves, as the site for this intense biochemical activity, are dense with vitalizing nutrients.

Vegetables generally have fewer calories and more nutrients and phytochemicals per forkful than any other food. These nutrition powerhouses, fundamental to the Perfect Formula Diet, have proven weight loss and health benefits.

- Vegetables fill your stomach with their high fiber and water content, but with exceptionally few calories. This characteristic helps you lose weight and keep it off.

- A Chicago study of 3,700 people ages 65 and older followed for six years found that those who ate the most vegetables best maintained their ability to remember, think, and otherwise function mentally.
- Men who eat the most vegetables have a lower risk of developing benign prostatic hyperplasia (enlarged prostate).
- A four-year study of more than 31,000 adults found those who ate the most salads and cooked vegetables had the lowest rate of diabetes.
- A wide variety of vegetables lowers the risk of developing non-Hodgkin's lymphoma, a type of cancer striking more people each year.

The next section outlines a few of the many studies combining fruits with vegetables to demonstrate additional, substantial health benefits.

Fruit: Why Humans Have Color Vision

Few animals have color vision. The fact that you distinguish and enjoy colors is an important clue about the foods you're designed to thrive on.

Ripe fruits are the most colorful foods in nature. Before people started buying food in grocery stores, even before the dawn of agriculture, foraging humans spotted colorful ripe fruit as a critical source of nutrients and calories.

Color vision was a key survival advantage for early people, precisely because fruit is an ideal food for humans. True hunters, such as dogs and cats, can't see in color because this would confer little survival advantage. Instead, these carnivores have super smell and hearing to aid them in spotting and tracking their prey. Recall that each species has those abilities that are most critical for its survival, based on the food it's meant to find and enjoy.

Plants produce fruit as a mechanism to spread their seeds. Since plants can't move and humans and other animals can, many plants rely on animals to eat their fruit and disseminate their seeds for the next generation. What a magnificent partnership nature has designed! The more tasty and nutritious a fruit is, the more enticing it will be to a hungry person or animal. Producing wonderful fruit has a survival advantage for plants.

You might have heard that fruit will slow weight loss because it's high in sugar. True, the carbohydrates in fruit are generally not as complex as those in many other parts of the plant, such as the leaves, stems, roots, or seeds. However, the sugars in fruit are bound in with a hefty amount of fiber, which slows digestion, controls blood sugar swings, and makes you feel full.

Fruit also contains an enormous amount of phytochemicals and other nutrients to signal your body's nutrition sensors that you should stop eating. Fruit has fewer calories per bite than most beans, potatoes, and whole grains.

Fruit, your Perfect Body, and your Perfect Weight were all made for each other. Anyone who compares the natural goodness of fruit, dense with countless nutrients, fiber, and phytochemicals, with manufactured foods, such as candy and cake, is forgetting about the basic principals of nutrition. A food can't be judged solely on the basis of the size of its carbohydrate molecules.

For purposes of the Perfect Formula Diet, fruit includes whole fresh or frozen fruit, not fruit juice. Fruit loses more than 90% of its nutritional components after being processed into juice. Thus, juice will not satisfy your nutrient sensors or help quell food cravings the same way whole fruit will.

When fruit is dried, most of the water in the original food is removed, so the fruit shrinks. On the Perfect Formula Diet, you are eating food based on volume, so dried fruit can be misleading.

If you eat dried fruit—such as raisins, prunes, dried apricots, dried figs, cranberries, and so on—eat only one third the volume you would eat of fresh or frozen fruit. So for example, if you're going to eat a cup of fresh fruit but substitute raisins instead, eat only a third of a cup of the raisins. Dried fruit will be less filling than fresh fruit because you eat a smaller volume. Eat most of your fruit as fresh or frozen, and keep dried fruit for a treat or for traveling. Chose canned fruit only if fresh, frozen, or dried are not available.

Fruit is a pillar of the Perfect Formula Diet:

- Fruit generally has more calories per bite than vegetables, but fewer than beans, potatoes, or whole grains. With this mid-range caloric density, plus a plentiful concentration of nutrients, phytochemicals, and fiber, fruit fills your stomach and turns off your appetite efficiently. A study of more than 100 people found that those who ate the most fruit had, on average, the lowest percentage of body fat.
- Fruit is colorful, appealing, and naturally delicious. Candy makers and bakers aim to capitalize on the great taste of berries, melons, and apples, but there's no way they can equal the incredible experience of eating ripe fruit.
- The availability of different kinds of fruit changes seasonally, ensuring you'll never be bored.
- Fruit is highly portable. Tuck several pieces into your purse, backpack, or briefcase for a filling snack wherever you go.
- Natural sweetness makes fruit ideal for a snack or dessert when you crave something sweet.
- Fruit is generally easy to digest.

In addition to fostering weight loss and sustained maintenance of your Perfect Weight, fruits boost your health so you can enjoy feeling and looking good. For example, a British study of 11,000 health conscious people found that those who ate fresh fruit every day had a reduced rate of death from heart disease, stroke, and all diseases combined.

Health studies often combine fruits and vegetables into one group when analyzing the impact of food on health. The lesson is to consume generous amounts of both kinds of foods.

- Eating fruits and vegetables fosters weight loss without hunger.
- Eating more fruits and vegetables leads to lower rates of obesity, even though people with this eating pattern tend to eat more food each day (as measured by the weight of food).
- The Nurses Health Study included more than 84,000 women, while the Health Professionals' Follow-Up study had more than 42,000 men. Putting results from these two massive projects together, researchers concluded that eating fruits and vegetables helped protect men and women from heart attacks.
- Fruits and vegetables nourish your brain, improving your mood and feelings of well being.
- In a recent study, eating more fruits and vegetables led to more minerals in the bones of teenage boys and girls as well as older women. However, the amount of calcium in the diet was not related to bone measurements for any age group.
- Fruits and vegetables help relax your blood vessels naturally, bringing down high blood pressure.
- The phytochemicals in fruits and vegetables protect your cells and artery walls from damage.
- Studies from all over the world consistently demonstrate that eating more fruits and vegetables helps prevent cardiovascular disease, diabetes, Alzheimer disease, cataracts, and cancer.

Beans, Peas And Potatoes: That Satisfied Feeling

Beans, lentils, and peas, known as legumes, are seeds from the pods of certain species of plants. Humans have grown legumes for thousands of years. Traditional diets worldwide include peas, soybeans, black beans, garbanzo beans (chickpeas), pinto beans, lentils, and many other legumes. The terms "beans" and "legumes" are often used interchangeably. However, "legumes" include peas and so is a broader category.

Have you been missing the incredible health, taste, and weight benefits of legumes? Then don't wait another day to start. Legumes are dense with nutrients, including minerals, protein, essential fatty acids, fiber, and numerous phytochemicals.

Scientists have studied soybeans more than any other legume. Phytochemicals called isoflavones act as weak estrogens in soyfoods. These isoflavones help enhance the effects of estrogen in your body when estrogen is too low, but weaken estrogen's activity when estrogen is too high.

Scare tactics about the feeble estrogenic effects of soy or any other plant are hype from animal food industries. Read Chapters 12 through 15 on health to learn about the far stronger estrogenic impact of female hormones in the milk of pregnant animals—otherwise known to you as dairy foods!

Studies have found that the isoflavones in soy have a beneficial effect on blood vessels, bone density, and kidney function; these substances may also inhibit the growth of cancer cells and act as strong antioxidants.

There's no reason to slight other legumes and focus on soybeans, just because this is where research is concentrated. Enjoy the full spectrum of colorful, tasty, versatile, filling beans, peas, and lentils. You don't need to eat soybeans at all if you don't want to.

There are so many excellent reasons that legumes play a major role in the Perfect Formula Diet.

- These foods are filling, digest slowly, and satisfy your appetite for a long period after you eat them.
- Legumes reduce blood sugar levels, assist in insulin control, and dampen food cravings.
- People who regularly eat beans weigh less, on average, than those who don't. Beans reduce the risk of obesity.
- Legumes are affordable and an excellent value for your food dollar.
- Legumes are convenient, usually available dried, canned, and sometimes fresh or frozen. Dried, frozen, and canned

beans and peas typically remain edible for months or even years after purchase, making it possible to stock up if you can't get to the store very often.

- Legumes boost your health. A four-country study of people over 70 found a 7% to 8% reduction in the risk of death from all causes for every additional serving of legumes eaten daily. In fact, legumes were the most protective food the elderly could eat. Beans also reduce cholesterol and the risks of breast cancer, enlarged prostate, and diabetes and they help normalize high blood pressure.
- Legumes favorably alter the bacteria in your colon, similar to the action of probiotics.
- The extensive variety of legumes provides a welcome range of tastes, textures, and colors for your meals. If you don't like one kind of bean, then try another. Eating tofu is not required, although it's definitely an option. If you prefer, you can enjoy garbanzos, green soy beans (edamame), black beans, pinto beans, white beans, red beans, kidney beans, lima beans, fava beans, peas, green lentils, red lentils, and many more.
- You can enjoy versatile legumes on their own, or in soups, burritos, casseroles, sandwich spreads, sauces, dips, salads, salad dressings, and many other satisfying foods.
- Legumes enrich the soil they grow in, contributing to a green and sustainable future for all.

Potatoes have only a few more calories per forkful than beans and also play a key role in the Perfect Formula Diet. People all over the world grow, love, and thrive on potatoes.

This important food has taken the fall for the high calorie and often unhealthy additives that may accompany it, including oils (for frying), butter or margarine for topping, and sour cream. Think of the evidence convicting potatoes of "making you fat" as purely circumstantial.

Potatoes have been framed. French fries and potato chips contribute to weight gain not because of the innocent potato, but because of oils and chemicals used in cooking them.

Actually, potatoes that are boiled, baked, mashed, or roasted without added oils or animal ingredients are quite healthy and should be a vital part of your weight loss plan. Choose baking potatoes, sweet potatoes, yams, Yukon gold, red, or purple potatoes, or any other varieties you prefer. Sample them all. Potatoes of different colors will have varied nutrients, so you benefit from eating many kinds.

Scrub your potatoes thoroughly and cook them unpeeled. Many of this food's healthy components are in the skin. Remember, nutrients turn off your appetite. So eating potatoes unpeeled will result in feeling full and satisfied with less food, and benefiting from additional vitamins, minerals, and phytonutrients. However, don't eat potatoes that have green discoloration under their skins or potatoes that have already sprouted, as these may contain concentrations of a harmful substance called solanine.

Here are the reasons the Perfect Formula Diet includes potatoes as an integral food.

- Potatoes are nutritious and are a versatile "comfort food" that will reduce food cravings for manufactured and animal foods. Potatoes are so healthy that people can thrive on potatoes if no other food is available.
- Potatoes will satisfy your appetite and reduce hunger better than just about any other food.
- Some people are not used to legumes and will take some time to accustom to their taste, adapt their digestive system, and learn to cook them. During this process, they can enjoy potatoes with about the same energy density as beans.
- Some people are allergic to beans, and may be able to eat legumes in limited amounts or not at all. Potatoes provide a ready alternative.

- Potatoes store well so you have to shop less often, and you can adapt them to many delicious uses. You can easily bring cooked potatoes with you when you travel.
- Baked potatoes are readily available in restaurants. Order a couple *without* butter and sour cream (use black pepper or other spices and salsa instead), and be prepared to leave the table satisfied and smiling.
- Potatoes thrive in harsh climates and make efficient use of farmland and other scarce resources, conserving the planet for our children's future.

Whole Grains: Now You Are Really Full

Whole grains, which are the seeds of certain grasses, are the fourth corner stone of the Perfect Formula Diet. Don't skimp on this foundation of appetite satisfaction and super nutrition because of phony hype or myths about grains or carbs.

These foods have been the basis of the human diet for more than 10,000 years, and groups of people who live mostly on whole grains are lean and healthy. Before grains were "domesticated" at the dawn of agriculture, humans undoubtedly ate the seeds of wild grasses—the ancestors of today's grains. These seeds would have been a key food for early humans. Otherwise, people wouldn't have bothered to figure out how to grow them deliberately.

People worldwide base their diets on wheat more often than any other grain, followed closely by rice as a top grain selection. Wheat berries can be cooked whole, cracked for bulgur wheat, or ground into flour for bread, pasta, cereal, and many other satisfying foods.

Brown rice is a whole grain; white rice is not. Oats (including oatmeal), corn, barley, spelt, buckwheat, rye, millet, wild rice, and quinoa are other delicious foods to round out the whole grain component of your diet.

Whole grains contain all parts of the seed—the bran (outer coating which protects the seed until it's ready to sprout), germ (the part that will germinate, or turn into a baby plant), and endosperm (food reserve for the baby plant). Refined grains, which are manufactured foods, contain only the endosperm.

In the refining process, grains lose critical fiber, vitamins, minerals, and phytochemicals, not to mention taste. If you're used to eating refined grains, then give your taste buds a few weeks to start loving the richer, more complex flavors and heartier, more satisfying texture of the entire seed.

How can you tell if a grocery product in your cart is whole grain or not? Here is a critical step you always need to take. Reading the label carefully is essential to ensure that some type of whole grain is the *first* ingredient in the list on the product. Many commercial foods masquerade as "whole grains," but really are not.

You're in for a pleasant surprise when you expand your diet to include more whole grains, as many have already discovered. One small study of overweight adults found that 9 out of 11 study participants preferred the whole grain diet tested over the study's refined grain alternative.

Whole grains are an essential part of your weight loss and lifetime weight maintenance plan.

- Whole grains make you feel full and satisfied simply because they contain enough calories to "turn off" your appetite and prevent, or at least lessen, food cravings. Whole grains also make your stomach empty more slowly after a meal or snack, so your hunger is turned off for a longer time. You'll find weight loss sustainable for a lifetime once you are no longer hungry.
- Whole grains, along with beans and potatoes, contain the least expensive foods on the Perfect Formula Diet.
- Whole grains can be familiar and delicious comfort foods. Substitute whole grains for many of the foods with refined grains you're likely eating now.
- There are a wide variety of whole grain textures and tastes, allowing you to experiment with new foods and expand your nutrition without getting bored.

- Whole grains, if stored properly, stay fresh a long time. This means you can stock up and make fewer trips to the store.
- Whole grains are portable. Think of a sandwich on whole grain bread or a small glass or plastic container of cooked whole wheat pasta, corn, or brown rice.
- Whole grains have the right number of calories to cushion your weight loss, which helps your liver keep up with the toxins dissolved in the fat you are losing.
- Whole grains make efficient use of farmland, producing impressive calories and nutrients per acre, often under harsh weather conditions. Of all crops, grains generally produce the largest amount of food per cultivated plot.

You might have been told that grains contain a substance called phytic acid which interferes with mineral absorption. Be aware of the whole story. This effect is countered when the grain is soaked, germinated, boiled, fermented, or otherwise cooked. Phytic acid is a powerful antioxidant which can reduce blood sugar, insulin, cholesterol, and tryglycerides.

Many people who think they are sensitive to gluten specifically, or grains in general, may in fact be reacting to refined grains or some unhealthy ingredient in foods made in factories.

Refined grains can cause blood sugar to spike and then fall as they are absorbed too quickly. Grains may be mixed in with animal foods, chemicals, and transfats in manufactured foods, or maybe you put butter or oil on whole grains yourself. These additives are the real culprits for most people, not the beneficial whole grain itself. If you think you may be allergic, give whole grains, healthfully prepared, another chance to see how great they can help you feel. You may find what you thought was a sensitivity to gluten evaporates into a non-issue.

About 1% of people do have true celiac disease and the gluten (one of the plant proteins) in wheat, barley, and rye triggers unhealthful reactions for them. If you have celiac disease, work with your health care provider to identify whole grains with low levels of or no gluten for the Perfect Formula Diet grain rotation. Rice is a safe grain for most people, as an allergy to rice is very uncommon.

Numerous research studies of the *actual* incidence of illness and risk factors among people on different diets find that whole grains, in practice, have a powerful range of weight and health benefits.

- People who eat more whole grains have a lower risk of being or becoming overweight or obese. The Nurses Health Study, which recorded information about more than 74,000 U.S. nurses for 12 years, found that the women who ate the most whole grains consistently weighed less than the women who ate the least whole grains and gained the fewest pounds over the study period. Another study of 285 adolescents found that the average BMI for teens who ate less than half a serving of whole grains a day was 23.6, but was a much healthier 21.9 for the teens who ate more than one and a half servings of whole grains daily.
- People who eat more whole grains tend to have lower cholesterol, blood sugar, insulin, and blood pressure.
- Whole grains increase your cells' sensitivity to insulin, which is a good thing because it then takes less insulin to properly burn glucose for fuel.
- Eating whole grains reduces the risk of many chronic diseases, including cardiovascular disease, heart failure, type 2 diabetes, stroke, and some cancers. In fact, a study of postmenopausal women found that eating as few as six servings a week of whole grains slowed the development of plaque build up in their arteries as much as treatment with statin drugs! A study of more than 86,000 male physicians followed for over five years found that those who ate the most whole grains had a 17% less risk of dying from any cause and a 20% reduced risk of dying from cardiovascular disease.

You can get a pound of organic brown rice for a little over a dollar, deliciously feeding both your stomach and your health for many meals.

Nuts And Seeds: Nutrient Packed Crunch

Nuts have a smaller role in the Perfect Formula Diet than other Perfect Foods, but still add welcome flavor, texture, variety, and nutrition. Because of their relatively high fat content, nuts have more calories per spoonful than most other Perfect Foods.

On the Perfect Formula Diet, you can eat a handful of nuts or seeds or a tablespoon or two of nut or seed butters four to six days a week. The nuts and seeds should be raw or dry roasted, not cooked in additional oils. Avoid nut butters with added oils, sugar, salt, or other ingredients that are not on the Perfect Formula Diet.

In addition, as described earlier, be sure to eat two tablespoons a day of *ground flax seeds* as your reliable source of sufficient omega-3 fatty acids, which will be in healthy balance to your omega-6 fatty acids, as long as you don't use manufactured oils. The flax seeds must be finely ground to break down the hard outer hull, which would otherwise impede their digestion. Store ground flax seeds in the refrigerator.

Walnuts are also a good source of omega-3 fatty acids. Researchers have found that walnuts lessen the damage to the inside of your arteries after you eat a fatty meal. Olive oil did not have this beneficial effect.

A study of more than 83,000 women found that those who ate a handful of nuts or one tablespoon of peanut butter at least five times a week were significantly less likely to develop diabetes than those who seldom ate nuts. Those Seventh Day Adventists who ate nuts five or more times a week cut the risk of having a heart attack in half.

Parsley: More For You Than Garnish

Herbs and spices are magic, transforming a plate of rice and beans or a bowl of split pea soup into a feast. Their enticing aromas indulge your sense of smell before you even begin to eat. Your taste buds leap with fulfillment. With this sensory gratification, you don't need to eat as much to feel totally satisfied.

By experimenting with the full range of herbs and spices, you'll keep your meals interesting and will look forward to Perfect Foods. You can rely on your current favorites and try out new tastes and aromas. You'll make food you'll be proud and happy to share with family and friends.

You may think you enjoy the taste of animal foods, but in fact you're not likely to get excited by plain boiled, unseasoned meat, fish, or chicken. You want your animal foods with herbs, spices, salt, sauces, smoke, dips, or other flavoring agents. By generously seasoning Perfect Foods with herbs and spices, you're less likely to miss animal foods and will transition more easily and happily to the Perfect Formula Diet.

Herbs and spices support good health as well as weight loss. Their dense flavors and aromas derive from potent phytochemicals that can fight inflammation, infection, and cancer, in addition to aiding detoxification, and protecting your cells. The nutrient-dense phytochemicals can also help turn off your appetite so that you need less food to feel full.

Herbs and spices are so powerfully beneficial that people around the globe have employed them as medicine for thousands of years. By consuming herbs and spices instead of salt, you'll cut down on your sodium intake, which may be helpful in controlling blood pressure and preventing osteoporosis.

Dark Chocolate: Thumbs Up

One of the easiest mistakes to make if you're eating the Perfect Formula Diet is that "a little bit" of animal food or manufactured food won't hurt, especially if you have a good excuse to eat it. Maybe you're at a restaurant with a client, and there's nothing obvious to order on the menu to fit your eating plan. Maybe it's a holiday and your former traditions are based on animal foods. Maybe it's your birthday, or your best friend's birthday, or your co-worker's retirement party. Maybe you're at your new neighbor's house for dinner, and they've cooked a meal with no Perfect Foods. Maybe you just had an argument with your spouse and are feeling a bit down.

The list of "maybes" is indeed endless. That's why "a little bit won't hurt" is such a dangerous idea to tell yourself. You undoubtedly know, from painful experience with past diets, that one "little bit" quickly leads to another and another, and soon your desired eating plan is history.

You can't negotiate with your body the same way you can with another person. Your Perfect Body really doesn't care *why* a harmful food just landed in your stomach. Excuses don't help either your weight or your health. The secrets to forestalling a "little bit" are to build commitment and establish new tastes and habits, which the rest of this book will jumpstart.

This said, it's unrealistic to think you'll never have another "special treat." The trick is to keep treats to small amounts, with no animal ingredients and minimal manufactured ingredients.

An excellent treat, rich in beneficial phytochemicals, is dark chocolate. Carefully read the label to make sure your choice is made without milk, butterfat, or other dairy components. You can eat half an ounce to an ounce of dark chocolate every day or two, or instead just eat two or three ounces of dark chocolate once a week.

Other acceptable treats, in small amounts a couple of days a week, are *100% plant-based* cake, cookies, or frozen desserts. If possible, aim for "junk foods" with some redeeming qualities, such as organic ingredients, unbleached flour, unbleached sugar, no chemical preservatives, and a lower fat or salt content.

Your occasional treats should never include any foods that are deep fried, or that are made with hydrogenated or partially hydrogenated oils, or that contain any animal ingredients.

Makes sure at least 95% of the calories in your diet come from Perfect Foods. In other words, if you were to consume 2,000 calories a day on average, or 14,000 calories a week, then no more than 700 calories a week (5% of the total) should come from your occasional treats. Rough estimation is fine.

Eat Your Calories, Don't Drink Them

Adequate hydration is necessary for survival, and your Perfect Body has intricate sensors to determine when you need more fluids. These are not the same sensors that determine if you need more calories or other nutrients. When you drink your calories, your body does not properly register this additional energy and still sends you out to eat food. So it's difficult to attain and maintain your Perfect Weight when you drink a significant number of calories.

For drinks, stick to water, sparkling water or club soda, white, green, black, or herbal teas, and an occasional cup of coffee (one or two cups a day), if coffee is part of your daily routine. Vegetable juices are generally low in calories, and you can have a glass a day of carrot, tomato, beet, or other vegetable or mixed vegetable juices.

Tea is an especially good drink choice because the beneficial phytochemicals in this beverage can protect your health and encourage calm, but alert, mental functioning. Be sure to drink good quality brewed tea, not a sweet tea-flavored manufactured substitute.

What if you're used to drinks that are sweet or flavored? There are two solutions to this problem.

The simplest is to recognize that your tastes will change. Although giving up soda, energy drinks, and fruit juice may initially be a challenge, after a period of a few weeks, you'll be used to the refreshing effect of water and tea on your body. If you then take a sip of your former favorite drink, it should taste too sweet and overpowering to you.

The second solution is to gradually change your drinks. Start by diluting fruit juice with a bit of water or sparkling water. Over a period of a few weeks, gradually increase the amount of water and decrease the amount of juice in each glass until you're down to about an ounce of juice diluted by eight to ten ounces of water or sparkling water. You can safely keep drinking juices that are diluted to this extent.

For "milks," there are numerous dairy-free choices made from soy, rice, oatmeal, or other grains, seeds, or nuts. Each type and each brand of these "milks" tastes different, so experiment to find the kinds you find most delicious. Some are flavored—vanilla, chocolate, even egg nog options. These dairy-free milks are great for cooking and for pouring over whole grain cereal.

You can lighten your coffee or tea with a small amount of dairy-free milk. If you're used to adding sugar, just gradually decrease the amount of sugar you add over time until you're down to none. Your taste buds will adapt. If you currently use artificial sweeteners, switch to the equivalent sweetness of sugar, then follow the directions above.

However, dairy-free milks are still a form of liquid calories, and you should limit yourself to no more than eight ounces a day if you want to lose weight. Once you're at your Perfect Weight, you may be able to add up to another cup a day and stay in maintenance mode.

Wine, beer, and other alcoholic drinks are loaded with calories that can separate you from your Perfect Weight. If you enjoy these drinks in moderation, experiment to see what works for you. One likely outcome is that a couple of glasses of alcoholic drinks a week are still compatible with an acceptable pace of weight loss. Any more, and you most likely would have to cut down on food to get to your Perfect Weight.

Skipping the food your Perfect Body needs in favor of drinking alcohol is a risky choice and definitely not recommended for your health—you could develop nutrient deficiencies. Plus alcohol can have serious health effects. Seek professional help if you have any question about your drinking habits.

Not Part Of The Perfect Formula Diet

The Perfect Formula Diet is free of meat, poultry, fish, eggs, anything made with or from the milk of another animal (designed by nature for babies of another species), vegetable oils in liquid form or margarine, hydrogenated vegetable oils, anything deep fried (such as fried potatoes or chips), protein powders, soda, energy drinks, and any artificially sweetened foods.

Stick to the amazing variety of appealing whole plant foods that you are encouraged to eat. You'll be happy you did.

Supplementing The Perfect Formula?

Plants are at the base of earth's food chain, which means that plants must manufacture the nutrients needed by either plants or animals. On the Perfect Formula Diet, you will eat abundantly of all the vitamins, minerals, and phytochemicals from these green factories. Supplements can upset the ratios of these healthful natural components to each other. How a nutrient works in your body is strongly influenced by the overall biochemistry of your body, not just the one factor in isolation from its surroundings.

The World Cancer Research Fund and American Institute for Cancer Research, in a 2007 report summarizing the result of decades of studies, concluded that high dose supplements can raise the risk of cancer in some cases. This is because the supplements may give you too much of a good thing. The report recommends that you eat a diet dense in nutrients from whole foods to assure your body is getting what it needs.

Another research overview of 68 studies, collectively including more than 232,000 people, focused on the health impact of vitamin supplements. After looking at the highest quality studies, the researchers concluded that people who took certain vitamins in supplements, including vitamins E, beta carotene, and A, had a higher risk of death than those who did not take supplements. The authors concluded you should get your nutrients from food.

Researchers tracking more than 300,000 men found that those who took multivitamins more than once a day were almost twice as likely to develop fatal prostate cancer as were men who never took multivitamins.

Each vitamin, mineral, and phytochemical has a role to play, and too much of one can keep the others from doing their jobs. Think of a sports team dominated by only one powerful player, who crowds out all his teammates and keeps them off the field. No matter how superb that mega-player, his team is not likely to shine in their games.

Two Nutrients Not From Plants

However, there are two nutrients your ancestors found in abundance that *are* in scarce supply in our modern world *and that do not come from plants.* Bacteria manufacture *Vitamin B12*, while your own body synthesizes *Vitamin D* from sunshine. You can think of this as a kind of photosynthesis that occurs naturally in your own skin.

On the Perfect Formula Diet, you need to take a Vitamin B12 supplement to make up for the fact that you are eating food and water that has been sterilized to kill just about all microbes. Buy a B12 brand that comes in a vegetable capsule (not a gelatin capsule), and follow the directions on the bottle or that your health care provider gives you.

Vitamin D is most problematic in winter, and in locations further from the equator. If you're not sure you're getting adequate sunshine then you may want to take a Vitamin D supplement. Again, buy a brand that comes in a vegetable capsule (not a gelatin capsule) and follow the directions on the bottle or from your health care provider.

Troubleshooting: You Can Do It!

If you're not losing a pound or two a week after a few weeks on the Perfect Formula Diet, or if you're not feeling at your best while on this diet, here are some possible reasons.

Not following the diet:

- *You are not eating the Perfect Formula Diet.* Be sure you're eating vegetables, fruits, beans and potatoes, and whole grains, each as one quarter of your food volume. Don't forget two tablespoons daily of ground flaxseed, and your B12 supplement taken as directed on the bottle. You may as well be honest with yourself. If the best you can say is that you are following the Perfect Formula Diet "most of the time," you can't expect optimal results. Even "a little bit" of animal or manufactured foods can sabotage your diet.

- *You are not eating enough food in total.* On the Perfect Formula Diet, it's critical that you eat when you're hungry and eat until you're full. If you skimp on food, you're cheating your body and the diet will not work properly. If you don't get enough calories, especially if you're physically active, your body will channel the nutrition it does get into its most vital functions, and other parts of your body will get shortchanged. If you don't have the appetite for larger meals, then make sure you eat numerous small meals or snacks throughout the day to get sufficient food. If you're doing intensive physical workouts, be sure to eat enough Perfect Food before, during, and after exercise to fuel your activity level. Otherwise, fatigue sets in and you may mistakenly think you need "more protein" or develop strong cravings for unhealthy foods.
- *You are drinking calories.* Switch to the drinks outlined earlier in this chapter. You may need to cut down on the dairy-free milks and cut out all fruit juices (even if diluted).
- *You are eating too many "junk food occasional treats."* Cut down on or get rid of these altogether, at least until you're at your Perfect Weight.
- *You are eating too many nuts.* Make sure you're eating no more than a handful or two of nuts four to six times a week, at least until you're at your Perfect Weight.
- *You are not reading food labels or not asking what is in your meals when you eat out.* You think you're eating the Perfect Formula Diet, but your assumptions about what's in your food are incorrect. For example, you may think you're eating whole grains, when in fact you're eating refined grains.

Another possibility is that your body is adjusting. This should be temporary.

- *Your body is detoxifying.* Stick to the Perfect Formula Diet and your body will bring the detoxification under control. Aim to eat organic food as much as possible, at least during this initial period when you are detoxifying fastest. That way your liver will cope with chemicals in dissolving body fat, but not the additional load of pesticide residues and other toxic components that might be in the food you are eating now.
- *You are withdrawing from animal foods and/or manufactured foods.* These types of foods have components that may be addictive. Again, stick to the Perfect Formula Diet, and the withdrawal symptoms will resolve themselves.
- *You have not properly adjusted the amount of prescription or nonprescription drugs, supplements, or insulin you now require.* Be sure to work closely with your physician in making these changes. Do not attempt to change any medication dosage or timing on your own. You may need to adjust the dosages immediately when starting the diet or several months down the road.
- *Your immune system and all the systems in your body are stronger and more responsive.* Why could this be a problem? Think of your immune system, on your usual diet, as an army of soldiers suffering from chronic fatigue interspersed with hair trigger over-responsiveness. If an enemy threatens, this army can react only weakly, or will overreact in a disorganized and ineffective manner. On the Perfect Formula Diet, your immune system is like a well trained army of Olympic athletes. The reaction to anything that could harm your body, including chemicals in your home, work place, cleaning products, personal care products, and so on, may be more pronounced. Signs this is happening may include cough, rashes, fatigue, or headaches. The chapter *Perfect Home* will help you ditch the toxic chemicals.

You may also react more forcefully to caffeine or other stimulants, resulting in a feeling of anxiety from an amount of coffee, or even tea, sugar, or chocolate that you could previously tolerate. The solution is not to purposely damage your immune and nervous systems with a bad diet, but to avoid the chemicals making you sick. Cut down the amount of these stimulants as necessary.

Other harmful habits may be hurting your naturally Perfect Body.

- *Other elements of your lifestyle choices are impacting your health.* While diet is the 800-pound gorilla in terms of determining your health, later chapters describe additional factors that can impact your health and weight. Included are sleep, air pollution, toxic chemicals, time in nature, and exercise. As you read these chapters, you can fine-tune your life choices to maximize health and weight loss.
- *You are smoking, using illegal drugs, or abusing prescription drugs.* You don't need this book to tell you how unhealthy these behaviors are. The Perfect Formula Diet cannot totally overcome the negative effects of smoking or drug use on your body. If you're having trouble stopping these behaviors, seek professional help. Many effective programs, some free or low-cost, are available to help you.

Another possibility is that you're not honoring your body's signals.

- *You're not sure when you are hungry and when you are not.* After years of eating manufactured and animal foods, and eating when external cues tell you to, you may have stopped paying attention to your body. If you need to feel what the hunger signal is all about, then go three to five hours without eating. When you start to eat after this, consume your food very slowly, and make sure you eat a balanced mixture of vegetables, fruits, beans and/or potatoes, and whole grains.

Pay attention to how the hunger signal weakens and fades. Stay focused on your body as necessary to reestablish communications with your natural signals.

- *You know you're not hungry but eat anyway.* You may do this because you're using food for emotional satisfaction or physical gratification. Work with a counselor, friend, or self help book to establish alternative ways to satisfy your emotional and physical needs. Make sure you eat only Perfect Foods.

- *You know when you're hungry but don't know or care when you're full.* This is a bit different from deliberately eating for emotional reasons or for the sheer pleasure of taste and smell. If you have this issue, you're probably eating fast, finishing off two or three large plates of food without even thinking about whether you're satisfied or not. Try eating very slowly, taking 15 or 20 minutes to finish one plate or bowl of food. Eat only one or two kinds of food at once, instead of a multi-course meal. Cut off eating after two cups of food, and don't eat again for a couple of hours, unless you actually feel hunger pangs. If you're still compulsively eating after trying these ideas, seek help from a counselor or program that specializes in eating disorders.

Please be patient with yourself. The Perfect Formula Diet becomes easier and easier the longer you stay on it. Upcoming chapters will give you numerous ideas to overcome potential obstacles as you experience a clear road to success.

Finally, following the Perfect Formula Diet can boost your health and energy but will not result in weight change if you're starting out at your Perfect Weight. Similarly, once you arrive at your Perfect Weight, you'll hold steady there.

The Story Condensed

Each of the pillars of the Perfect Formula Diet is necessary and beneficial. While you can have an occasional "junk food treat" (dark chocolate being most recommended), you need to pay attention to what you drink as well as what you eat. Issues to resolve spring from not consistently following the Perfect Formula Diet, detoxification and withdrawal from prior food choices, other harmful habits, and not honoring your body's signals. Each of these issues can be resolved.

The Perfect Formula Diet moves "balanced" into the 21st century, leaping to excellence and eclipsing run-of-the-mill diets. With the Perfect Formula Diet, you're balancing groups of Perfect Foods, each with its own characteristic caloric density, nutritional profile, phytochemicals, tastes, textures, aromas, shelf life, and costs, in order to achieve a whole that is more than the sum of its parts. If this appeals to you, read on to learn how to jumpstart your new food choices and strengthen commitment to your powerful, effective eating plan.

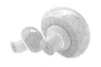

CHAPTER 8

Perfect Start

You can think of your choice this way. Which would you rather do:

- Follow the Perfect Formula Diet now and weigh four to eight pounds less at the end of the month; or
- Eat as usual and, at the end of the month, weigh the same or more, feeling the same tight waistbands snug around your body?

How much of a lifestyle change are you willing to make to permanently achieve your Perfect Weight? Would you be willing to move to another city? Change careers? Get married or divorced? Would you be willing to start speaking a new language, make all new friends, or take a vow of silence?

The good news is that it's not necessary to do anything nearly so radical to live at your Perfect Weight. *In fact, you really don't need to do much.* All that's required is to upgrade your food choices to nature's finest offerings and eat to satisfaction when you're hungry. Is that really so hard?

You may be feeling ambivalent about a major change in your diet, no matter how desirable. Such nagging uncertainty is normal with any significant decision, even when the benefits are clear-cut.

Realize that certainty follows behavior, not the other way around. When you begin eating the Perfect Formula Diet, your thoughts and attitudes will slowly but surely morph to support your new choices.

To successfully launch better food selections, you'll benefit by planning for three areas of thought and action:

- Commitment: your consistency in making the Perfect Formula Diet work for you
- Strategy for your transition: completely following the Perfect Formula Diet right away or evolving gradually from your current eating patterns
- Logistics: shopping for, cooking, and eating Perfect Foods (this is the fun part)

This chapter supports you in building commitment and thinking through your transition, while the next chapter addresses logistics.

Several of the ideas in this chapter incorporate short writing exercises. Jotting down a thought strengthens it and gives you the opportunity to think through what you really want. So you'll benefit from getting a small notebook for your Perfect Formula Diet ideas and observations or creating a folder on your computer to keep your writings together.

Establishing Commitment

Commitment is the bedrock of success. Logistical concerns, such as what to eat for dinner or how to figure out food ingredients in restaurants, all have practical answers that become second nature over time. But to find and use these solutions, first you must build a foundation of dedication to making the Perfect Formula Diet work for you.

Initially your commitment doesn't have to be that high. The Perfect Formula Diet intensifies its own commitment and momentum when you stick to it, because you'll feel healthier, vibrate with energy, lose weight, and experience success. You'll find that logistical barriers melt in the heat of commitment, so your determination will strengthen over time.

Think about how good you felt the last time you succeeded at something important. Form a mental image of that personal triumph and journey to that memory. You probably felt strong and able to do it again and again. Write a short description of that experience. This is how you'll feel after you've been on the Perfect Formula Diet for a couple of months. The ideas in this chapter aid you in establishing the initial commitment to get that far.

Solidifying Commitment

As the Perfect Formula Diet transforms your weight and health, you can discover even more reasons to solidify your commitment to this eating plan. In addition to feeling and looking better, on the Perfect Formula Diet you'll enjoy food more—the subtle, intricate, natural flavors and textures of Perfect Foods. Your senses will brighten as your eyes, ears, and skin finally receive all the nutrients they need, and toxins are eliminated.

You'll feel closer to the beauty of nature and to your companion animals. Your food choices will parallel the highest ethics and values. You can enjoy each meal as a celebration of life.

As you succeed on the Perfect Formula Diet, you'll feel more in control of your life in other areas and generally more hopeful and optimistic. As the quality of your life rises, stress becomes more manageable.

Commitment is a choice—your choice. You are committed no matter what, either to business as usual or to a meaningful change. Which will you select? Choice is a responsibility you can't escape. Your decisions reverberate far beyond your own health—to your family, friends, acquaintances, and in fact to all living beings on the planet.

So state your commitment out loud, to yourself, and to others. Write down why you will be consistent and what your goals are. Then share your thoughts with family, friends, or co-workers.

Commitment And Confidence

Confidence that you can succeed dramatically enhances your ability to succeed. Every positive experience of the Perfect Formula Diet strengthens your self-assurance. Each time you cook a good meal, dine out and stick to your eating plan, or try a new fruit or vegetable, you build your foundation of hope and confidence.

Think of an activity in which you're very confident of your skills. For example, you may know you're good at car repair, reading, computer games, a sport, singing, knitting, training your dog, or any other skill that comes to mind. Think about the first time you ever performed this activity. How confident were you then? How did you build your confidence and expertise until mastery was second nature? Write down your answers.

Then think about the Perfect Formula Diet. The same growth of confidence and self-assurance in eating Perfect Foods is there for you when you cultivate it. Commitment and confidence develop together, and the good news is that each reinforces the other.

If possible, find a friend, co-worker, or family member to share the Perfect Formula Diet with. Teaming on this eating plan will spur your success as you and your food partner learn and grow healthier together.

Questions Are Good

Your new food choices may draw questions from family and friends. Many of the queries will be friendly and curious. This is an excellent opportunity for you to strengthen your resolve by educating others. Most people don't need detailed information. All you need to do is assure them you're eating nature's finest foods and avoiding foods that will harm your health. Simply say you are on a whole-foods plant-based diet and are getting the optimal amount of protein, vitamins, and minerals.

As you lose weight and gain energy, people are sure to give you compliments. This is another opportunity to let them know you're happy with your new choices. The more often you tell people about the Perfect Formula Diet in a positive light, the more your own commitment will solidify for the long term.

Enlist the aid of family, friends, or roommates. Ask for their support in keeping animal foods and manufactured foods out of your life. Tasty food is your best weapon in this process. Many people will be won over when you share samples of your favorite recipes.

Keep asking questions yourself. Be your own scientist. You don't need to believe what's in this book or any other single source of information. To the extent that you can understand the jargon, study medical textbooks and articles in reputable journals. Always be on the lookout for media hype, and delve into conflicting studies you see in magazines or on television to discover limitations in the research and its funding. Never accept headlines at face value.

Be willing to question your own former beliefs. After all, science is about advancement and discovery. At one time, "experts" agreed that the sun revolved around the earth, that the earth was flat, that germs had nothing to do with disease, and that second-hand smoke was safe. Don't get left behind as knowledge advances!

Most importantly, observe yourself and others. How do you feel when you consistently follow the Perfect Formula Diet, especially after any initial detoxification period is ended? What happens to your weight? How does this compare to what you've experienced on previous diets?

A few people may openly oppose your new choices, either out of misinformation about nutrition or anxiety provoked by your success. Some people feel threatened by anyone who makes choices different from their own. You'll gain little by arguing with such people. Your success is the best answer to their concerns. Once you give them some general facts and refer them to this book or another source of scientific discussion, your job is done. While you can explore various tactics, the one most likely to work is simply to change the subject and talk about something besides food.

Take Advantage Of Your Curiosity

You've likely tried numerous name-brand diets before and none has worked long term. This experience may have left you with a deep sense of disappointment or defeat.

As you've read through this book, you've probably realized that you didn't fail the other diets. Instead, *those diets failed you.* The long list of over-hyped diets you attempted worked against your body instead of with it, leading to inevitable poor results.

Are you curious to find out what it would be like to follow an eating plan that works with your naturally Perfect Body? Would you want to be the first to bring such good news to your family and friends? Give your curiosity freedom to check this plan out.

Keep Taking Notes

Writing down your reasons to follow the Perfect Formula Diet and tracking your successes are excellent ways to build commitment and guide your choices. Here are some ideas.

- Make a list of your top three goals for the Perfect Formula Diet. For example, you may want to improve your energy, be more attractive, or set a good example for your family. You may want to take your dog for longer walks, accomplish more on the weekends, or have no part of factory farming. Come up with your list and post it where you'll read it frequently. Make your reasons *specific*. For example, the goal of "normalizing blood pressure to 120 over 80 without medications" is more compelling than a general goal to "improve health." "Fitting into size 6 pants" is a better reason than simply "losing weight."
- Read your top three goals out loud to yourself frequently and edit or expand the list as you think through your goals. Visualize your achievement of each goal in detail.
- Write affirmations on a regular basis to support your confidence and build commitment. For example, you could

put on paper or softcopy into your computer, "I am losing weight," "I am succeeding on the Perfect Formula Diet," "I am learning to enjoy cooking," or any other affirmation that is helpful to you. Write for five minutes a day.

- Keep track of what you eat. This will help you identify problems (for example, you're not eating enough vegetables) and reinforce your success when you make good choices.
- Make a list of your favorite recipes that are consistent with the Perfect Formula Diet.
- Track your weight. Be sure to weigh yourself in the same clothes (or no clothes) and at the same time each weigh-in. It's best to weigh yourself only once a week as your weight will fluctuate a bit from day to day. Make a chart as your weight goes down, and put it somewhere prominent—you earned the right to be proud of yourself.
- Track your other health risk factors, such as blood pressure and cholesterol, as these improve.
- If your doctor tells you it's okay to stop taking a medication you used to need, put the empty pill bottle in your bathroom or on your bedside table as a reminder of improving health.
- Keep a record of the money you're saving through any reduced need for drugs or medical care and by avoiding increasingly expensive manufactured and animal foods. You can buy yourself or a family member a gift with these savings or donate the money to your favorite charity. You can also "fine" yourself if you don't follow your eating plan.
- Pay attention to strategies that build commitment for you. What thoughts, feelings, activities, and images strengthen your resolve to work with your Perfect Body? Write these down and reread them whenever you need to.

It's All In Your Attitude

You have the power to take any feelings of deprivation and actively reframe these as liberation, a challenge, an adventure, or anything else that feels positive to you. Deprivation is truly a function of your attitude, and if you are not in control of your attitude, who is?

We all make food choices every day. Most of us chose not to eat bugs, garbage, or cat food, even though we could if we wanted to. We don't see this self-imposed dietary limitation as constricting, because we don't see insects or pet food as anything we would want to eat. You can cultivate the same attitude about manufactured and animal foods.

At first you may find the Perfect Formula Diet to be inconvenient, but convenience has many dimensions. Weighing in above your target weight, having to constantly shop for new clothes as your weight fluctuates, spending time at the doctor's office and the pharmacy, having trouble with daily activities because of chronic pain—all these possible consequences of your current diet are even more inconvenient, aren't they? As you develop new habits and master the logistics of the Perfect Formula Diet, the convenience factor will fade away.

Before starting the Perfect Formula Diet, you may be anxious that you'll miss your old favorite foods. In reality, your tastes will change within a few weeks. You won't miss animal foods and manufactured foods nearly as much as you anticipate. This is a basic survival mechanism. When your ancestors were foraging for food in nature, they had to be willing to eat what they found. If they held out for foods not available, they would have starved.

Make a list of and find or draw pictures of Perfect Foods that you really enjoy. If there were no advertising, who would choose an oily, salty, unnatural chip over a colorful, exquisite bowl of freshly cut, juicy pineapple or watermelon?

You think you eat foods because you like them. But the reality is the reverse. You like foods because you eat them. Once you're on to this secret, you're only a few weeks away from finding that Perfect Foods are your new mealtime and snack favorites.

Rediscover the pleasure of real food, not packaged, greased, overcooked, processed, bleached, deodorized, chemically preserved, oversalted, and oversweetened, but Perfect Food as it comes from the fields and orchards. Encourage your taste buds to revel in what this food tastes like, smells like, and feels like.

Change Takes Time

Change doesn't usually happen all at once, nor does it follow a straight line. As long as you're taking more steps forward than back, you are getting somewhere. Be patient with yourself as you adopt the Perfect Formula Diet.

Success is its own reinforcement. Every day that you feel better, you'll want to feel better still. You'll naturally keep raising the bar for yourself until you can sense that time is running in reverse. Take advantage of the magic of this process.

Focus on the current moment and determine which of the five stages of the change process you're in for adopting a new eating pattern.

- Precontemplation: you're not aware of the change or interested in making it. Since you're reading this book, you're probably past the precontemplation stage.
- Contemplation: you're simply thinking about making a change.
- Preparation or decision: you're actively planning for a change you want to make.
- Action: you're in the process of carrying out a desired change.
- Maintenance: you're through all the initial stages and are sustaining and building on the positive changes you have accomplished.

Think of a change you've successfully made in your life. What motivated you to make this change? What old beliefs and activities did you need to modify in order to transition?

Think about it and write it down. Add to your thoughts over time. Apply what you discover to moving on to the Perfect Formula

Diet. Write down what it will take to get you to the "action" stage of change and why you want to get there.

Two Paths For Your Future

Your Perfect Start can follow either of two paths: a gradual, systematic transition or a swift transformation in your food choices. Either decision is valid, with its own advantages and disadvantages. If you're in a hurried or acutely stressful phase of life, or if you're early in the stages of change outlined above, you might elect a more gradual start. You'll do best if you assess and honor your feelings.

Success in losing weight and improving health goes up *dramatically* when you follow the Perfect Formula Diet *completely*. While a slow transition is a valid choice, if that's what you decide on for now, have realistic expectations. If you follow the Perfect Formula Diet only occasionally and incompletely, your resulting weight loss and health improvement will be modest, at best.

Once you're following the Perfect Formula Diet consistently, you'll see a *dramatic* change in your ability to eat to satiation while still attaining and maintaining your Perfect Weight. Depending on your health issues, you may also experience a very substantial improvement in your health, mood, and energy level.

Major shifts in eating patterns are easier for many people to follow than are small changes. When you totally revamp your foods, your taste buds change their preferences within a few weeks. If you continue to eat your old favorites, even in small amounts, your old tastes are still being nurtured.

If you find a small change in diet daunting, you may jump to the conclusion that a larger change would be even more difficult. However, a small change has modest payback, while a major transition puts you into a new, sustainable set of habits with gratifying rewards.

With a little practice, you may find the Perfect Formula Diet easier to follow than a limited version of your current diet. For example, 35 women followed a whole-foods plant-based eating plan as part of a study on menstrual symptoms. Only three out of the 35 said it would be difficult to follow the plant-based diet after the study, and more of the women liked the study diet over their usual diet.

Here are some ideas to help you plan your strategy.

- Realize that on a typical diet, you may develop an addiction to some of the proteins, stimulants, and chemicals in animal and manufactured foods and that you may go through some withdrawal symptoms when you start basing your diet on Perfect Foods. A gradual transition can help stave off symptoms of withdrawal and detoxification, and you may find this helpful. On the other hand, how long do you want to delay the detoxification process? Your withdrawal symptoms from addictions to unhealthy foods resolve when you *totally* stop eating the addictive substances.
- Wipe out preconceived ideas of what will be difficult or easy. Allow yourself to be surprised by how simple the transition can be. Your nutrient deprived body will soak up Perfect Foods the way the thirsty summer earth soaks up water.
- Once you do begin the Perfect Formula Diet in earnest, the improvements you feel are so significant that virtue becomes its own reward. On the other hand, modest changes in your eating are not as self-reinforcing, because you won't notice as much in the way of weight loss or improved health as a result. You'll get out of the Perfect Formula Diet exactly what you put into it.
- A gradual transition is a valid path as long as you have a plan to track your progress. Write down what you eat and how you feel after you eat. Make a list of your successes, even if it's just one meal based on Perfect Foods. You'll build momentum over time, even if you don't expect to.

So grab hold of your life and go for success on any level you choose. Write down the results you want, give yourself a timeline, and track how you're doing every day. Whichever path you choose, get started. Even small changes will move you nutritionally toward the ideal. The worst thing you can do is—nothing!

You Are Going In The Right Direction

Simply by reading this book and learning fact-based nutrition, you are forging ahead. This is a big step. You're doing what is right for you and your family.

If you do stray from the Perfect Formula Diet, there is no point in beating yourself up. Simply note what you have learned and start with your new eating plan again. You didn't learn poor eating habits overnight and it will take some patience to build the Perfect Formula Diet into an effortless routine.

If unmanageable food cravings, binge eating, or other eating disorders persist after you have consistently followed the Perfect Formula Diet for several weeks, seek help from a health care professional. Eating disorders are dangerous health conditions that require specialized treatment.

Down Payment On The Rest Of Your Life

A helpful resolution to the gradual vs. swift transition issue is to commit totally to the Perfect Formula Diet from day one of your change, but mentally frame the transition as a month-long commitment.

This month-long shift is not a "cleanse" or any kind of permanent cure for weight or health issues. The toxins in your naturally Perfect Body accumulated over decades and can't be eliminated in a few weeks or even months of some short-term "cleanse."

The most accurate way to think of this month-long trial is as a down payment on the rest of your life—a down payment whose value is always there for you. Unlike money you may put toward buying a house or car, you can't lose the value of your initial commitment to the Perfect Formula Diet.

If you choose to stay on this eating plan long term, then you've taken a giant step toward your Perfect Weight and health improvements. If you decide to go back to your usual way of eating, you'll have demonstrated to yourself that you can follow the Perfect Formula Diet with noticeable results and may opt for a longer trial or permanent commitment any time you want.

Staying Balanced On The Surfboard

Maintenance is an *active* phase of change and as important as accomplishing the first triumph of success. You're at risk if you don't consciously sustain the good you've achieved for yourself.

Have you ever watched surfers riding waves? Think about how long the surfer stays balanced on his board, riding the incalculable power of the ocean. As long as the surfer moves forward, he or she usually remains standing and enjoys the ride. As the wave slows, the surfer starts to lose balance and inevitably falls once the board loses its forward momentum.

This observation has everything to do with success on the Perfect Formula Diet. Keep moving forward and you can keep your balance as long as you want. Get into a static mode and your chances for long term success diminish.

You don't need to advance forward every day, but several times a week is helpful. Think about all the fun ways to stay positive and focused on continuing success. Small actions are enough to keep you on your surfboard. Here is a sampling of ideas:

- Talk to a friend, neighbor, co-worker, or family member about your success
- Write and rewrite your list of reasons to eat the Perfect Formula Diet
- Read and reread sections of this book and make notes about your insights and ideas
- Search out new sources of recipes that are based on Perfect Foods
- Prepare new recipes and share these with your friends, family, or co-workers

- Try new herbs, spices, and other Perfect Foods
- Find a meal at a new restaurant that fits into the Perfect Formula Diet
- Search out different websites, books, and magazines related to reasons for eating Perfect Foods
- Join an online group of people whose diets are based on plant foods
- Shop at a new health food store or supermarket
- Take a cooking class that teaches you how to prepare tasty meals from Perfect Foods
- Attend a potluck or dine out where most people will be bringing or ordering dishes made from Perfect Foods
- Go to a seminar or lecture, or even a residential program, focusing on the importance of eating whole plant foods
- Watch a video about factory farming, global warming, or the health benefits of Perfect Foods
- Reread the first section of this chapter to keep the changes you're making in perspective
- Volunteer to be of service to your local community
- Visit an animal sanctuary to get to know and bond with animals

You may be skeptical that raising money for a homeless shelter, tutoring a child who needs help with reading, volunteering at the local humane society, fostering a litter of abandoned kittens, or writing a letter to the editor about global warming will help you stay on a healthy diet. Yet each will take you outside yourself and your narrow concerns, focus you on the future, and put your actions in a larger context. All these choices, along with thousands of other positive activities you will come up with, keep you moving forward to maintain your balance and momentum on the Perfect Formula Diet.

The Story Condensed

The next month will come and go, and you are in control of what you will accomplish. A change in one area of lifestyle—eating—will lead to major rewards. If you choose to stay on the Perfect Formula Diet, your commitment and confidence will naturally blossom with your success. You can enhance this process with strategies to solidify commitment.

You can follow either of two paths: a gradual, systematic transition or a swift transformation in your food choices. Either decision is valid, with its own advantages and disadvantages. One effective option is to follow the Perfect Formula Diet consistently for a month as a down payment on the rest of your life. At the end of the trial period, evaluate and decide your next steps.

If you stagnate on the Perfect Formula Diet, chances are you'll revert to your former eating habits sooner or later. Keep up your forward momentum by deliberately making positive choices to try new foods, share and build your knowledge, and help others several times a week.

CHAPTER 9

Perfect Logistics

You already plan your meals and snacks, but this process may be largely unconscious and repetitive on your usual diet. If you generally eat the same foods every week, shop in the same stores, and frequent the same restaurants, you don't really need to spend much time mapping out the process.

When your diet changes, however, you start to think about what you will eat, where you will buy it, how you will cook it, and how you will assure that Perfect Foods are available when you are hungry.

Create your own convenience. The ideas in this chapter and the additional tools in Chapter 21, *Perfect Resources* will give you a head start on success.

Don't worry. The longer you stay on the Perfect Formula Diet, the easier planning becomes. After a while, eating will go back onto automatic pilot once you have figured out what works for you. Commitment will get you through the early stages, when choices are not yet familiar and second nature. After that, eating will be no more challenging or time consuming than it ever was before.

Have fun with this planning process. Enjoy the colors, textures, tastes, and aromas of new foods and fresh recipes. Savor every victory over weight-promoting choices as you reeducate your taste buds. Relish that your body feels younger every day.

Shopping For Perfect Foods

Shopping can be a pleasurable adventure, the next best thing to plucking Perfect Foods from your own garden.

- Explore the Perfect Foods in your local grocery stores where you are used to the layout. Notice how colorful the produce section is. Buy at least one kind of fruit or vegetable you have not eaten in a while (or ever).
- Pay attention to foods you may have overlooked, such as soymilk, rice milk, soy yogurt, whole grain pasta, brown rice, or intriguing spices. Taste treats such as plant-based burgers, edamame (green soybeans), miso (a tasty fermented soy paste that makes terrific soups), and soy- and rice-based frozen desserts open a new world of healthy alternatives.
- Plan your shopping list and buy food when you aren't hungry. You'll make less impulsive purchases.
- Keep out of the chip and soda aisles, and avoid the meat, fish, chicken, dairy, and egg departments.
- Try shopping in new venues, such as natural food stores and farmers markets, which are exciting alternatives to traditional supermarkets.
- Depending on where you live, flax seed (an essential part of the Perfect Formula Diet) may be difficult to find in either whole or ground form. You may also not have much of a selection of dairy-free milk substitutes. Check out the Internet to supplement your store purchases, as necessary.

You'll soon learn which of the thousands of food choices are delicious and healthy. Your shopping trips then become shorter and routine.

- Roughly plan your eating for the week before you shop and make a list of the Perfect Foods you'll need. Many whole grains, beans, potatoes, spices, dried fruits, and frozen foods store well, so don't be afraid to stock up. Fresh fruits and vegetables do best when eaten soon after purchase, so you may need to do occasional quick stops just for fresh foods. You can supplement with frozen foods in between shopping trips.
- Read *all* labels until you learn which specific products fit your plan. *Reading labels is your best protection against foods that will undermine the Perfect Formula Diet.* Look for plant ingredients, whole grains, minimal or no added oils, low sodium, and no hydrogenated or partially hydrogenated vegetable oils. If a label lists any animal ingredients (such as meat, fish, chicken, eggs, egg whites, cheese, whey, casein, milk in any form, gelatin, and so on), hydrogenated or partially hydrogenated vegetable oils, or chemicals with long names leave the product on the shelf. The "mystery" ingredients are probably not anything you want to eat.
- Products made with small amounts of white flour, liquid oils, or added sugar or salt are in a gray area. These kinds of foods may be okay for a special treat or an occasional convenience, but minimize their use in favor of Perfect Foods. Usually the last items the label lists are the ones used in smaller amounts.
- For grain products, the first ingredient should be a type of *whole* grain, such as whole wheat or brown rice. "Wheat flour" and "unbleached wheat flour" are *not* whole grains.
- When you're first starting the Perfect Formula Diet, emphasize potatoes rather than beans for that category of foods. As your digestive system adapts to beans, you can start revising the ratio to reflect more beans and fewer potatoes if you choose.
- Experiment with different brands and flavors of dairy-free milks until you find one or two you really enjoy. You can choose from soy, almond, hazelnut, oat, hemp, and rice milks.

- Experiment with different brands and flavors of veggie burgers and other prepared "meat substitutes." You can enjoy these in limited amounts while you discover whole plant foods to eat instead, since the more manufacturing, the less healthy.

To the extent possible, don't watch, look at, or listen to food ads. These ads are designed to manipulate your craving for unhealthy, but highly profitable, manufactured and animal foods. Realize that three quarters of the new foods inundating stores are candies, condiments, refined grain breakfast cereals, drinks, refined flour baked goods, and dairy products—just about nothing of interest for the Perfect Formula Diet.

The Perfect Formula Diet Comes Home

Home cooked meals are the yummiest part of the Perfect Formula Diet, but you don't need to be a master chef to turn out tantalizing food. Prepare fragrant recipes so your house smells delightful and enticing.

You can join the swelling ranks of people rediscovering the joys of cooking from scratch. The more time you spend shopping for and preparing home-cooked meals, the more likely you are to be a healthy weight.

- Unless you love cooking and have lots of time, keep most of your meals simple. Herbs and spices make meals tasty, and don't require long and elaborate cooking techniques. Fresh foods retain their appealing textures, aromas, and tastes when lightly steamed, sautéed, or roasted to perfection.
- To avoid using manufactured oils or margarine, "stir fry" foods in a little water, vegetable broth, juice, or wine instead. Keep adding more liquid as you stir fry, so there is always some in the pan.
- On weekends or when you have time, prepare larger quantities of food and freeze the leftovers. When preparing for

dinner, aim to cook enough to have leftovers for lunch the next day or two.

- Experiment with your current favorite recipes by modifying them for the Perfect Formula Diet. For example, white spaghetti with meatballs and an oily or cheesy sauce may morph into whole grain spaghetti with a tomato-based sauce with no added oils. Use beans, lentils, baked tofu, and/or steamed vegetables for the toppings, and sprinkle on lots of herbs and spices.
- If you never enjoyed cooking before, start with simple recipes or take a few cooking lessons. Cooking is creative, relaxing, and gratifying. You can listen to music or podcasts or talk on the phone with a friend while you cook. You may be amazed to find you enjoy cooking far more when you're working with colorful and appetizing Perfect Foods. We can't all be farmers or even gardeners, but we can all work with food from the land.
- Soup is the ideal food for the Perfect Formula Diet. In many soups, you create a one-pot tasty marriage of beans, peas, or lentils, with potatoes, vegetables, and whole grains, flavored generously with your favorite herbs and spices. You don't have to be overly precise in cooking soup. If you put in too much of something, you can usually dilute the effects with more water or vegetable broth. If you don't add enough of something, you can correct that as well. Serve your soup while it's hot, so you'll eat it slowly. This gives your digestive system's nutrient sensors time to register what you're consuming and you'll naturally eat fewer calories.

Here are some more effective food preparation tips.

- Cooking is more fun if you prepare meals with a family member or friend.
- Savor the wait for delayed gratification as your food cooks. Instant food may be okay, but you miss the anticipation of

waiting for something wonderful and the reward when it sits temptingly in front of you.

- Keep your house stocked with large amounts of Perfect Formula Diet staples, such as herbs and spices, canned and dried beans, frozen and fresh fruits and vegetables, potatoes, brown rice, whole grain breakfast cereals, dairy-free milk, and oatmeal.

- Find recipes for Perfect Formula Diet foods on the Internet or in cookbooks and have fun experimenting. See Chapter 21, *Perfect Resources* for ideas. If you don't like the result, eat a little bit anyway. Your tastes will adapt over time.

- Invest in kitchen equipment to make cooking faster. Even something as simple as a good garlic press or rice steamer can make your life easier. Your health is worth it.

- Watch out for salad dressings (this is true regardless of where you are eating). You may be enjoying the world's healthiest salad in terms of Perfect Foods, but if the salad dressing is made with oil, milk, cheese, sour cream, or other animal or manufactured foods, you are wiping out most of the good inherent in the salad.

See what strategy works best for others in your household.

- If you're choosing the Perfect Formula Diet and others in your family aren't, then they can eat what you're eating and supplement it with whatever unhealthy additions they insist on. There's no need to cook two totally separate meals.

- If possible, keep animal foods and manufactured foods out of your house—if you have any on hand, give them away if possible, or at least keep them out of sight in an inconvenient location.

- Initially, you may need to spend additional time planning and working out food arrangements with your spouse, partner, kids, roommate, or whoever shares your kitchen or meals.

Don't expect those in your household to immediately start eating like you, or even to be supportive of your efforts. There's no benefit to lecturing or persuading others to join you in this new way of eating or to stress yourself out about the desires of others. Simply let them observe you happily serving as a role model, give them information if they request it, and have Perfect Food available for them if they want to sample your choices.

Prepared foods, such as canned soups and frozen veggie burgers and dinners, may supplement your home cooked meals as needed. As a general rule, cook your own food from scratch as much as possible, even if it's just lentils and steamed vegetables with paprika or fresh garlic on a whole grain tortilla.

Most prepared foods are expensive and are made with too much oil and salt. Researchers videotaped 32 families with two working parents preparing meals. This study found that packaged convenience foods didn't save time in preparing meals. Instead, the pre-prepared foods just substituted for simpler meals the family would otherwise have made from fresh ingredients.

Graze when you're hungry, rather than waiting until "mealtime" when your appetite has gotten out of control. If you follow the Perfect Formula Diet by including a series of small snacks or mini-meals, instead of three large, predetermined meals a day, you won't miss the loss of animal foods as the "entrée" for lunch or dinner.

Eat slowly and truly savor the beauty of Perfect Foods. Feel yourself connect to our great planet with every bite. Imagine the peacefulness of the fields and orchards where your food grew, and focus on these mental pictures while you cook and eat.

Reread Chapter 6 periodically to make sure you're following the Perfect Formula Diet. A key part of your strategy is to eat when you're hungry. Make sure you're not trying to artificially limit portions or calories and that you're eating the recommended categories of food in the suggested proportions.

The Perfect Formula Diet Goes To Work

Instead of unimaginative lunches or greasy fast food, brighten your work day with Perfect Foods. Contrast the flavorful, abundant foods you enjoy during the day with your co-workers' likely more scanty and less tasty meals and snacks. You'll feel privileged to be eating the Perfect Formula Diet.

If your workplace doesn't have a refrigerator or microwave, is it possible to get these installed? Band together with a few co-workers and ask your manager. When you're not preparing your own food, stay out of the kitchen, lunchroom, or anywhere else that people leave unhealthy temptations for their co-workers.

Here is how to get happily through your work day.

- Bring lots of Perfect Foods to work—enough for all the meals and snacks you think you might want. You can always bring the leftovers home or save them for the next day.
- If you're usually rushed in the morning, pack your lunch and snacks the night before.
- Invest in an insulated bag in which to pack your lunch and snacks.
- If you can, put up photos of colorful fruits and veggies in your workspace.
- Instant oatmeal is a wonderful snack. It's filling, inexpensive, and requires only hot water and a cup or bowl. Make sure there are no animal foods in the oatmeal, and look for brands with low sugar content per packet. You can also make your own instant oatmeal out of regular oatmeal. Simply put the oats into a blender or food processor and grind very briefly. Experiment with small quantities until you get the results you want.
- Canned soups with Perfect Food ingredients are another handy snack. Think black bean, split pea, lentil, or vegetable soups. Keep a can, can opener, bowl, and spoon in your workspace and heat the soup in the microwave if you didn't bring in quite enough food to get you through the day.

- Baked potatoes are another excellent and portable snack, as is fruit and cut up vegetables, such as carrots, celery, peppers, and cucumbers.

Also pay attention to what you drink.

- Bring a mug and tea into work and enjoy tea as you hit any rough patches during the day.
- If you must drink coffee at work, bring a small container of dairy-free milk for creamer (never use "nondairy" powdered creamers as these are manufactured foods, and most actually contain dairy proteins).

The Perfect Formula Diet Eats Wherever

Eating out is fun and you can master any initial challenges.

- If you have any say in the selection of a restaurant, choose one that you know has at least one meal based on Perfect Foods. Ethnic restaurants, such as Chinese, Thai, Indian, Vietnamese, Mexican, Middle Eastern, and Italian usually have rice, beans, pasta, and vegetables you can order right off the menu.
- Often cheese or sauces can be left off a standard menu item at your request, resulting in a dish that meets the Perfect Formula Diet guidelines.
- Ask your server to check with the kitchen if he or she is not sure about the ingredients in a menu item.
- If you can, call the restaurant before going there or check out its menu on the Internet. If there are no menu items that are consistent with the Perfect Formula Diet, request in advance that the chef prepare a special creation for you. Most restaurants are eager to satisfy their customers, and chefs love being freed from the confines of a fixed menu. You don't need to feel you are inconveniencing anyone when you have a special request.

- If you are at a restaurant that doesn't have Perfect Food choices, and you didn't have time to call ahead, simply put in your special request when you order. Chances are you'll have the best meal at your table because the cook will put some thought and creativity into it.
- Enjoy the fun of checking out promising restaurants you haven't tried before.
- Order water or herbal or green tea with your meals instead of other beverages.

Travel benefits from some planning.

- If you're traveling, scope out promising restaurants before you leave home by searching on the Internet for Chinese restaurants, Italian restaurants, vegetarian restaurants, farmers markets, natural food stores, and similar choices at your destination. You don't need to limit yourself to this list, but you'll feel more confident of your options as you travel.
- When you're on the road or at your destination, check the Yellow Pages or ask the locals about healthy eating options. Supermarket salad bars may have healthy and inexpensive options consistent with the Perfect Formula Diet.
- When you travel, keep a supply of portable healthy snacks, such as fruit, soy jerky, and whole grain cereals or crackers with you.

Enjoy meals with your family and friends.

- If you're eating at a friend or family member's house, bring a Perfect Formula Diet food choice with you. If at all possible, let your host know your food preferences in time to incorporate them into meal planning. If your host cannot or will not make a dish consistent with the Perfect Formula

Diet, then still attend to be sociable, but either eat the food you bring, eat before you go, or eat after you leave.

- If you don't know what the food choices will be, or if they will be limited, simply eat before you go to the restaurant or friend's house, and when there eat just a small salad or some other non-filling Perfect Food item. If you're pleasantly surprised at the restaurant by an appealing full meal choice, order the best option and take the leftovers home. At a friend's house, simply enjoy smaller portions if you have eaten before the meal.

- Meals are a social occasion. You don't need to miss out on the fun because you are on the Perfect Formula Diet. In fact, as you feel better and lose weight, your social options will grow. Simply learn to ignore what your family or friends are eating, and enjoy their company independently of food. Anyone who truly cares about you will be delighted at your soaring health and shrinking waistline, and their friendship will not depend on your food choices.

- Find plant-based meet ups or potlucks in your community by asking your friends, natural food store employees, healthy restaurant servers, or by searching the Internet.

Be ready to compromise your food choices to some extent when you're in a situation with limited selections. For example, you may need to eat white pasta instead of whole wheat, or white rice instead of brown. Your food may be cooked in oil and have too much salt. You may have to eat one food category (such as whole grains or potatoes) multiple times in a row before you can rotate to one of the other Perfect Food types (such as fruit).

It's almost impossible to avoid these dilemmas on occasion. Set firm boundaries for yourself. White pasta and white rice are okay for an occasional meal out, but animal foods, deep fried foods, chips, soda, and foods cooked in hydrogenated vegetable oils *never* are.

Avoid the mistake of thinking your food choices don't matter when you eat out or travel. They do. Remember, your Perfect Body doesn't care who cooks the food or why you're eating it. When you fall into the trap of "just this once doesn't matter," then success may elude you. Plan in advance and *be consistent,* and you'll get the results you want.

Start New Traditions

You may have traditions in your family or your culture of eating certain animal foods or manufactured foods at special holidays or other celebrations. Certainly it's important to honor these customs, which connect past and present and make you feel grounded in your community.

All traditions had an origin and evolve over time, so you're free to inaugurate new ones. Your new traditions will connect you with the future, as well as the past and the present.

For example, think about Thanksgiving. Your current tradition probably centers on turkey and includes potatoes, stuffing, cranberry sauce, vegetables, salads, and pies. It's easy to build on this tradition and establish a new custom of eating everything but the turkey, or substituting a non-animal look-alike for the turkey. In recent years, sales of turkey-free entrees have soared at Thanksgiving.

The Story Condensed

At first, the logistics of the Perfect Formula Diet may seem challenging. Commitment will carry you through until this way of eating becomes easy, second nature, and your first choice. The actions for getting to this point are straightforward:

- Plan for eating at home and out.
- Enjoy new foods, different recipes, and new grocery stores and markets. Be open to the best that nature offers you, and Perfect Foods will become your new favorites.

- Relate to people instead of foods when you get together with family and friends.
- Remember who is in control—you are!
- Be patient with yourself and others, have fun with the process, and savor every bite of Perfect Foods.

Everything else is detail.

CHAPTER 10

Perfect Price

Animal foods and manufactured foods are heavily advertised because of their profitability to their producers. When you buy such items, you pay a hefty premium that generates those profits. How often do you see ads for unprocessed Perfect Foods such as broccoli or black beans? On the Perfect Formula Diet, you can buy food like a budget-savvy expert and eat better than royalty.

Certain fresh fruits and vegetables may *seem* more costly than bulk cartons or bags of manufactured foods. When you look at value—nutrients and health outcomes—per dollar there is no contest. *Perfect Foods always trounce the competition.*

Perfect Foods deliver the most nutrition per dollar spent. A food that makes you overweight and sick is *never* a bargain, even if it's free.

On the Perfect Formula Diet, you eat regular food—forget the expensive prepackaged meals of some name brand diet programs.

Perfect Foods On A Budget

Unprocessed or minimally processed beans, potatoes, and whole grains are among the most inexpensive foods. On the Perfect Formula Diet, half of your food intake will be these bargain powerhouses.

As for the other half, carefully selected fresh or frozen fruits and vegetables don't need to break your budget. And while herbs and spices may seem expensive, remember you need only tiny amounts. A small jar of a spice may last for several months to a year, depending on how often you use it.

Here are some ideas to keep your costs down on the Perfect Formula Diet.

- For Perfect Foods that can be stored a long time without spoiling, such as dried or canned beans and lentils, potatoes, oatmeal, brown rice, dried fruit, and frozen fruits and vegetables, stock up when there's a sale.
- Buy in bulk whenever possible. Natural foods stores usually have bulk sections for foods such as nuts, flax seeds, dried beans, pasta, dried fruit, oatmeal, rice, and flour. Some stores sell spices in bulk as well.
- Buy fresh fruits and vegetables when they're in season to avoid higher priced out-of-season offerings.
- Comparison shop among farmers markets, supermarkets, membership or warehouse stores, and natural food stores to learn which ones have the best deals on specific foods. Some chains, such as Trader Joe's, have a large selection of Perfect Foods at lower prices than many natural foods stores or supermarkets.
- If you can get a better deal buying a large amount of something (such as a several pound bag of apples) and it's more than you need, split the cost and food with a friend or neighbor.
- Eat simply. Meals and snacks don't need to be elaborate to be satisfying and delicious.
- Tasty, inexpensive peanut butter and jelly sandwiches are probably one of your favorite foods. The Perfect Formula Diet encourages you to enjoy this pleasure—just make sure to use animal-free whole grain bread and peanut butter with no preservatives, chemicals, or added oils.

You can save money by doing things yourself.

- Grow some of your own food, even if it is just herbs on a windowsill or balcony.
- Preserve some of the food you grow or buy in season or in bulk. Take a class to learn how to safely preserve food while retaining as many nutrients as possible. Many foods can be frozen with no special method required except to seal them in airtight containers or bags. To preserve by drying, you can use your oven or purchase a dehydrator.
- Grind your own peanut butter or other nut butters.
- Learn to make your own soymilk, rice milk, and nut milk.
- Bake your own whole grain bread using a bread maker as a short cut. Once you smell and taste homemade bread, the packaged varieties will pale in comparison.
- Join or start a co-op, a food store owned by shoppers and/or employees. Such stores aren't profit-driven and frequently offer excellent prices. Or you could join a buying club, which is an association of individuals who pool their purchasing power. Search the Internet and see Chapter 21, *Perfect Resources* for more on buying clubs in your area.

Save Your Money For The Good Stuff

Another way to keep costs down is to not buy what you don't need. At the top of this list should be supplements. Except for vitamin B12 and possibly vitamin D if you have limited access to sunshine, you don't need to spend money on routine supplements. Likewise, stretch your budget by not purchasing gimmicky foods and drinks that have been reinforced with mega-doses of vitamins, minerals, or other nutrients.

Remember, your power team is an array of Perfect Foods, dense with thousands of nutrients and phytochemicals assembled by nature in the exact proportion your naturally Perfect Body will thrive on.

You'll also spend less when you bring lunch to work instead of eating out. As your cooking skills improve, you'll enjoy preparing your own food and will be happy to save restaurants for special occasions.

Cook in bulk and freeze leftovers for homemade frozen lunches and dinners—you'll conserve time as well as money. Save convenience foods, like frozen pre-made dinners from the grocery stores, for when you truly don't have time to make your own meal. Just be sure to buy animal-free choices.

Even when you travel, you can often bring some of your own food or buy fresh Perfect Foods in a local grocery store or market, thus saving on eating out, as well as preserving your health.

When you're lean and healthy, you're less likely to lose wages from being out sick. Your productivity will soar and your work life will become more profitable and successful.

As your health improves, the chances are excellent you'll save significant sums on prescription drugs and medical costs. However, don't discontinue or change the dose of any medication except with the supervision and consent of a health care provider.

The Story Condensed

The Perfect Formula Diet can easily be the most economical way to eat. Figure out how to make Perfect Foods fit your food budget. You can stretch and expand that budget by eating at home, bringing your lunch to work, taking food when you travel, leaving most supplements on store shelves, and eliminating any medical services and drugs that become unnecessary as your health problems fade.

Invest in your and your family's lean weight and optimal health. How could you better spend your money? If there are higher priorities for your purchases than Perfect Foods, you might want to volunteer at a hospital, hospice, or nursing home to see what happens after a lifetime of eating manufactured and animal foods. You'll help those in need in your community and reinforce your own sense of what's really important at the same time.

CHAPTER 11

Perfect Evidence

Every participant in any research project is a human story. As you read study results, think about cancer patients not as numbers, but as people with worried families and interrupted lives. You can picture chronic disease averted as 10 years of good life, visiting with family and friends, filled with pride at a grandchild's graduation, realizing a lifelong dream of that long trip to Europe. Then the numbers will talk and you can hear their message.

Studies of what people eat in their usual lives, outside of limited research settings, bring nutrition down to earth. By seeing what groups of people eat and how lean and healthy they are as result, you can conclude which patterns of eating are best.

The information this chapter presents is compelling evidence that the Perfect Formula Diet is based on the best foods on earth while excluding foods that researchers find harmful. On the other hand, if you have little interest in nutrition studies, feel free to skip to the next chapter.

The Nutrition "Controversy" Trap
You can stay out of the media-based "controversy" trap by understanding that science is about the weight of evidence, not perfection. Not all research is equally valid. The best studies are well-designed,

thoughtfully executed, and carefully analyzed. However, no single study is flawless or sufficient in itself to solve nutritional puzzles. Anyone can take a sliver of a study, based on faulty reasoning or even a statistical fluke, and generate a finding to say anything (even that smoking is beneficial to your health!).

Such pitiful "evidence" shows only the bias of the researchers or their big-money industry sponsors, not real world insights. If you pay attention to the weight of high quality studies and your own critical thinking, you'll have the best guidance.

After all, our bodies work a certain way and no amount of speculation, industry-paid studies, or wishful thinking can change the actual facts. So there's no reason to shrug your shoulders and give up on finding reliable answers.

Research in the U.S. is a $55 billion a year industry with big-money sponsors whose financial well-being is on the line. In an endeavor this massive, problems, biases, and errors are bound to occur. So look for clear-cut and consistent patterns of evidence.

Measuring Two Things At A Time

Scientists, like anyone else, appreciate convenience. Simple studies are the frozen, microwavable dinners of research—reliable, well-accepted, easy, and often a short-cut for something that could be far better. In studies that focus on only two factors, scientists hone in on one thing they can measure, which could be vitamin C, calcium, fat, blueberries, fish oil, or just about anything else. The point is to use statistics to "isolate" this factor and see how it's connected to a limited number of outcomes, such as colds, heart attacks, asthma, cancer, longevity, obesity, or endurance.

Most of the studies this book discusses fall into this category of simplified studies because the vast majority of nutritional studies of humans use this research method. While the findings have some value, the importance of the *pattern* of what people eat and other elements of their lifestyle gets lost. Moreover, statistics can be manipulated so the findings mirror the original bias of the researchers and their sponsors.

Since the human body is so complex, simplistic studies can go only so far in getting you the answers you want. Nutritional theories are most compelling when many scientists have all found the similar results.

In looking at popular studies in the media, watch out. A U.S. Department of Agriculture study of more than 16,000 people found that about two thirds of those who considered themselves "vegetarian" actually ate meat, poultry, or fish at least once during the two days before the survey. Look for studies that reliably measure what people actually eat, not what they say they eat.

The Full Pattern Gives You The Best Solution

Some research studies are more valuable than others. Epidemiology is a method that clarifies the occurrence of human diseases in a variety of countries and settings. Such research follows people in their everyday lives. The results paint the big picture for you so you can feel confident that you are making the best food choices to stay healthy and slim.

Complex epidemiological studies are expensive, time-consuming, and challenging, which explains why there aren't more of them. You'll benefit from the findings of two landmark epidemiological studies:

- The China Study: Dr. T. Colin Campbell's well-known massive probe into eating patterns and health in China in the 1980s
- Seventh Day Adventist nutrition and health: An intensively studied religious group that recommends a meat-free diet and healthy lifestyle as spiritual discipline

Some China Study Highlights

The China Study, which the *New York Times* called "the Grand Prix of epidemiology," capitalized on a one-time opportunity to explore on a grand scale how food choices relate to what illnesses people get—or don't get. This research was conducted in China in the 1980s, when most Chinese lived in the same location for a lifetime and ate, of necessity, local foods.

More than 90% of the participants in the China Study lived in the same area in which they were born. This lack of mobility created an unparalleled living lab to test how dietary patterns over a lifetime impact health.

Dr. Campbell, along with colleagues from Europe and China, gathered comprehensive information on diet, risk factors, and illness from 6,500 adults in 65 rural and semi-rural counties that spanned China. The researchers took blood tests and collected urine, directly measured all the food the participants ate, and analyzed food samples in the local marketplaces. This level of detail and data validation is rare in research studies, which often rely on participants' recall of what they ate or food diaries that may or may not be accurate.

The China Study participants ate a predominantly plant-based diet, although there were significant differences across regions. On average, animal protein supplied only 1% of their calories; the level in the U.S. today is about 10 to 12 times that percentage. The average China Study participant had a cholesterol level of 127 and some groups had average cholesterol levels as low as 80.

Dr. Campbell determined that eating animal foods led to higher cholesterol levels, and eating plant foods led to lower cholesterol levels. *He found animal protein (including protein from fish) raised cholesterol more strongly than saturated fat and dietary cholesterol.*

More China Study Findings

The China Study highlights can help you understand positive vs. risky eating choices. You get to select, to a large extent, what illnesses you will suffer over your lifetime.

- After adjusting for body weight, the Chinese consumed about 2,641 calories per day while Americans ate 1,989—yet the Chinese had only a fraction of the U.S. obesity level. Higher exercise levels in China did not explain this difference.
- The death rate from heart disease was 17 times higher in the U.S. than in rural China, while the death rate from breast

cancer was five times higher among U.S. women than among Chinese women.

- Participants in more economically developed areas, who ate more animal foods and oils, tended to develop "diseases of affluence," that plague developed countries. Such illnesses include colon cancer, lung cancer, breast cancer, leukemia, diabetes, coronary disease, and brain cancer in children. Cholesterol levels strongly predicted who would suffer from these diseases of affluence in China.
- Poor participants in rural areas developed "diseases of poverty," including pneumonia, intestinal obstruction, peptic ulcer, nephritis, tuberculosis, other infectious and parasitic diseases, and rheumatic heart disease. These poverty-stricken people may have lacked adequate food or eaten spoiled, contaminated, or improperly fermented food.
- Participants who ate even small amounts of animal foods tended to suffer a significant increase in chronic degenerative diseases.
- Those with more antioxidants in their blood tended to have lower cancer death rates.
- Plant protein worked as well as animal protein in assuring children achieved their maximum growth potential. Children's growth was stunted by overall lack of food, monotonous diets, poor public health, and high rates of childhood illnesses.
- Even though the Chinese consumed few dairy products and had an average calcium intake of 544 mg per day, their hip fracture rate was only about one fifth as frequent as the rate in Western countries.
- Even small amounts of animal foods caused measurable negative health effects, including higher cancer rates.

For a complete and engrossing description of this critical research, read *The China Study* by Dr. T. Colin Campbell.

A Real World Meat-Free Group

The Seventh Day Adventist denomination, started in 1863, includes about 13 million members. This religion emphasizes a healthy life-style for spiritual reasons and forbids alcohol, tobacco, and some biblically prohibited foods such as pork.

Going even further, this denomination recommends regular exercise, avoiding meat (including poultry and fish), coffee, tea, highly refined foods, and tongue-burning spices. Adventists in the U.S. choose to follow a range of food choices. About 3% are on an animal-free diet, 27% are meat-free but may eat dairy or eggs, and 20% eat meat less than once a week.

Researchers in multiple countries have intensively studied thousands of Adventist members because of their demonstrably superior health and long life spans.

- Adventist men have a significantly reduced risk for heart disease, cardiovascular disease, and stroke compared to comparable non-Adventist men; this is true even adjusting for tobacco use.
- Adventists under the age of 75 have lower rates of cancer and are less likely to die from cancer if they do develop it—this is true even looking only at tobacco-free non-Adventists. Researchers attribute the differences mainly to diet.

Researchers have learned much by contrasting specific Adventist eating patterns.

- Adventists who ate the least fish had a lower risk of prostate cancer; those who drank the most milk had the highest risk of prostate cancer.
- While those who ate red meat doubled their risk of colon cancer, those who ate fish and chicken tripled their risk of this diagnosis. On the other hand, eating beans more than twice a week reduced the risk of colon cancer by half.

- Adventist women who ate cheese at least three times a week had 43% higher risk of developing breast cancer than did their fellow church members who ate cheese less than once a week.
- The more meat a member of this community ate, the more likely he or she was to be obese.
- The risk of suffering a fatal heart attack increased by up to 50% for Adventists who ate meat once a week or more.
- Adventists who ate more fruit had a lower risk of lung, prostate, and pancreatic cancer.
- Meat-free Adventists were substantially less likely to suffer from diabetes, high blood pressure, arthritis, and other chronic diseases than were their meat-eating counterparts. Not unexpectedly, the meat avoiders used substantially less prescription drugs than Adventists who ate meat.
- *Adventists on a totally animal-free diet had lower cholesterol and blood pressure than their counterparts who ate dairy foods and eggs.*

Adventists are among the longest-lived groups ever studied.

- Male Adventists, on average, live five to nine years more than their non-Adventist counterparts, while women live two to five years more.
- Meat-free Adventists live, on average, two years longer than Adventists who choose to eat meat.

For the Adventist subgroup that was a healthy weight, avoided meat (including chicken and fish), and exercised, the common causes of death were delayed 12 to 14 years for men and 9 years for women.

More Observations Of Animal Foods

Epidemiological evidence abounds on the negative health effects of animal foods. These findings are based on research in which different people ate widely varying amounts of such foods. Here are some studies from specific countries that experienced significant changes in diet.

- In Scandinavia during World Wars I and II, people had to virtually cut out eating meat because of shortages and restrictions. During those times, death rates plummeted and people lived, on average, an additional two years. After the wars, the death rate soared as people began to eat meat again.
- In Japan, the rate of breast cancer jumped after the Japanese began eating more like Westerners. In the 50 years from 1947 to 1997, and adjusting for age, the death rate from breast cancer doubled and from ovarian cancer quadrupled. During those years, the amount of milk in the Japanese diet increased 20 times over, meat intake went up 10 times, and eggs eaten went up 7 times. In this same timeframe in Japan, the rate of testicular cancer also soared and the death rate from prostate cancer increased 25-fold.
- For Japanese women, the death rate from breast cancer increased more in wealthier socioeconomic classes, those who could most afford the Westernized diet of meat, eggs, milk, and fats and oils.

Other studies examine how health varies with diet across many countries.

- A study of prostate cancer mortality across 32 countries found the strongest risk factor for death from this cancer was eating animal foods.
- Two studies of breast cancer in 42 countries found that the amount of meat eaten—followed by milk and cheese intake—was most closely correlated with how many women developed this disease.
- A study across 42 countries found that cheese was the food most closely linked to the rate of testicular cancer in young

men, and that milk had the strongest link to prostate cancer. Rates of testicular cancer are highest in countries that consume the most milk and cheese.

- International studies have discovered that eating more dairy products is associated with higher rates of hip fractures and eating more animal fat is associated with higher rates of breast cancer, bowel cancer, and heart disease.
- An analysis of 34 hip fracture studies from 16 countries found a higher rate of hip fractures in countries in which people ate the most animal protein.
- Other epidemiological studies indicate that eating more animal protein is associated with accelerated growth rates, earlier sexual maturation, and increased risk for many kinds of cancer.

How Much Evidence Do You Need?

Researchers demonstrate again and again the effect of eating animal foods on health. Here's a tiny sample of additional real-world observations on cancer.

- Prostate cancer. A study of more than 82,000 men followed for eight years found that men who drank the most low fat or nonfat milk had an increased risk of prostate cancer. Researchers followed 20,000 male physicians for 11 years and observed those who ate the most dairy products had a 32% higher risk of prostate cancer. Epidemiological studies have observed that dairy products, red meat, and total dietary fat increase the risk of developing prostate cancer.
- Non-Hodgkin's lymphoma. Looking at 832 women with this diagnosis, researchers concluded that eating animal protein every day led to a higher risk of developing this type of cancer. Those who ate the most animal protein had a 70% greater chance of getting this disease.
- Breast cancer. A study of more than 23,000 women aged 50 to 64 in Denmark found that women who ate the most fish,

regardless of the type of fish or how they cooked it, had a 47% higher breast cancer rate.

- Endometrial cancer. In examining the diets of more than 2,400 women in China, researchers found that women who ate the most animal protein had twice the risk of developing endometrial cancer.
- Ovarian cancer. An overview of 12 studies that encompassed more than 553,000 women concluded that women who consumed the most lactose (the sugar in milk) had the highest risk of ovarian cancer.
- Bladder cancer. Two studies enrolling more than 170,000 people found that eating bacon frequently and eating chicken without skin were associated with a significantly higher risk of developing bladder cancer.
- Liver cancer. A study of 9,221 adults concluded that eating a diet high in protein significantly increased the risk of liver cancer (and also cirrhosis).

Other studies of the effects of animal foods on other illnesses are no more encouraging:

- Hip fracture. Women who ate the most animal protein in relation to the amount of plant protein had almost four times the risk of hip fracture.
- Alzheimer's disease. A study of almost 3,000 Japanese-American men living in Hawaii found that those with higher estrogen levels had a greater chance of developing Alzheimer's disease. Animal foods are the main dietary source of estrogen.
- Parkinson's disease. A study of more than 130,000 men and women concluded that those who consumed the most dairy products had a 60% greater risk of developing Parkinson's disease. Another study of 7,500 men in the Honolulu Heart Project

found that drinking more than two cups of milk a day more than doubled the chance of developing Parkinson's disease.

- Arthritis. A study of more than 25,000 adults in Europe found those with the highest protein diets had almost triple the risk of developing inflammatory arthritis.
- Diabetes. Looking at more than 37,000 women, researchers found that those who ate the most animal protein had a 44% higher risk of developing type 2 diabetes.
- Heart attack. Mercury enhances the risk of heart attack and fish is the main source of mercury for most people.
- Overall rate of death. About 23,000 people in Greece were observed for more than 10 years. Those who ate the most protein relative to the amount of carbohydrates were 70% more likely to die during the study period. Another study found that eating seven or more eggs a week was associated with a 23% greater risk of dying.

Perfect Foods And Cancer

Science supports a diet based on Perfect Foods. After reviewing a mountains of evidence, the World Cancer Research Fund recommended that people eat a diet based on unprocessed plant foods, including vegetables, fruits, whole grains, and legumes, to minimize the risk of cancer. An unending stream of specific studies supports this conclusion. Just a few examples include:

- Onions, other vegetables, and cereals strongly reduced the risk of death from prostate cancer in multi-country studies.
- The closer prostate cancer patients stuck to an animal-free diet, the more their PSA levels went down and the more effective their blood grew in killing prostate cancer cells.
- A study of women in 40 countries found that eating cereals and legumes was protective against breast, ovarian, and endometrial cancers.

- Looking at more than 800 non-Hodgkin lymphoma patients, researchers observed that cruciferous vegetables, tomatoes, onions, leeks, salad, and citrus fruits all reduced the risk of developing this diagnosis.
- Dietary flax seed slowed tumor growth in women with breast cancer.

More Views Of Perfect Foods

Looking outside of China, Dr. T. Colin Campbell concludes that chronic illnesses, which he calls diseases of affluence, are almost unknown in societies that eat mostly whole plant foods. Additional studies support the specifics.

- Pinto beans lower total cholesterol and LDL cholesterol.
- Eating fruits and vegetables leads to higher bone mineral density, helps maintain muscle mass in older men and women, and is protective against chronic diseases including cardiovascular disease, heart attack, stroke, diabetes, Alzheimer's disease, cataracts, inflammatory bowel disease, asthma, rhinitis, and cancer.
- An animal-free diet helped women conquer menstrual pain and gain energy.
- After just 11 days on a plant-based diet, men and women saw their cholesterol decrease by an average 11% and their blood pressure fall by 5% to 7%.
- A plant-based diet improved joint stiffness and pain for fibromyalgia and rheumatoid arthritis sufferers.
- Whole grains tend to lower blood insulin levels, systemic inflammation, and the risk for coronary heart disease, diabetes, and some cancers.

Think about the following impressive findings.

- After four weeks on a whole-foods plant-based diet, men and women enjoyed significant reductions in blood pressure, cholesterol, triglyceride levels, and glucose levels. Many were able to cease taking medications for chronic illness.
- A study of more than 32,000 men found that those who ate the most vegetables and legumes were the least likely to develop benign prostatic hyperplasia (BPH), while other studies reinforced the importance of eating vegetables to ward off this uncomfortable condition.
- In two studies, men who ate ground flax seed saw their PSA and cholesterol levels decline significantly. Flax seed also reduced the rate at which prostate cancer cells grew.
- Walnuts help blood vessel walls function better after a high fat meal.
- Nuts and seeds are associated with lower levels of the inflammatory markers CRP and IL-6.
- Proteins from plants lower the risk of high blood pressure.
- Researchers who studied three groups of exceptionally long-lived people around the world concluded by advising people to eat a healthy and varied plant-based diet.

While a discussion of all the studies showing the health effects of Perfect Foods would overflow any book, this sampling will give you a feel for the awesome benefits. *Talk about consistency—just about every study ever done of Perfect Foods finds something to praise. Now that's science—and food—you can feel good about.*

The Story Condensed
Industry-funded studies that manufacture "controversy" need not confuse you about the consistent weight of scientific evidence. Epidemiological "real world" studies are your most reliable source of nutrition information.

The China Study, Seventh Day Adventist research, and piles of additional studies all clearly and consistently demonstrate the superiority of a plant-based diet for smashing obesity, preventing disease, and adding healthy years to your life.

Since no single study is flawless or definitive, you will do best to follow a diet that many studies find health-promoting and few find harmful.

If you hold out for absolute "proof" of every principal of human nutrition—in the sense that there is not even one dissenting study—you are likely to wait until you lose the fun in your life to disabling illness, spend the money you saved for your grandkids on prescriptions, and wake up in intensive care. You can do better than this!

CHAPTER 12

Perfect Health

Getting to your Perfect Weight would not do you much good if getting thinner made you sick. And what if you're already at an optimal BMI of 20 to 23 and weight is not an issue. Can you still benefit from the Perfect Formula Diet while maintaining this Perfect Weight?

As the studies in Chapter 11 show, the Perfect Formula Diet should result in substantial improvements in your health while you lose weight. Perfect Foods can aid in preventing and reversing chronic disease, even if weight is not an issue for you. Don't miss the gratification and quality of life that Perfect Health brings.

Read on to gain a deeper understanding of why the Perfect Formula Diet can have such a dramatic and beneficial impact on your health, regardless of your weight. This diet book, unlike many others, does not present a simplistic picture of how your body works. Instead, you will find out about some critical bodily processes and hear about studies that indicate how these complex processes may be lined to weight and health.

Why Drunk Driving Is Illegal

If you're driving under the influence, you're not guaranteed to get into an accident. If you're driving sober, you still might not arrive safely at your destination. So why is drunk driving illegal, and rightly so? Because driving under the influence greatly increases the *likelihood* that you will get into an accident.

Having health risk factors is similar to drunk driving. You may have lots of risk factors and live to be 90. Or you may have no risk factors and not make it past 40. Still, look at the likelihood of achieving the result you want. *Risk factors are as undesirable for a healthy, independent long life as drinking is for a safe drive home.* As you read about health, keep this basic concept in mind.

What's Going On Here?

If you have a medical condition expected to last a year or longer, then you have a chronic disease. High blood pressure and arthritis are the two most common chronic conditions in the U.S.

If you have a chronic illness or frequent pain, watch out! Countless studies warn that you're likely to get sick with an additional malady.

The tendency of one chronic illness to lead to or be packaged with others is so common that it has a scientific name: "multimorbidity." In published medical studies, "multimorbidity" is shorthand to indicate that a person has several medical conditions at the same time. ("Multi" means "many" and "morbidity" means "illness.")

The frequency of multimorbidity is slippery to measure, because some groups of people are more likely than others to experience this unfortunate condition. Also, various researchers count specific chronic conditions as an "illness" while others use a different definition.

One finding is universal: the older you get, the more likely you are to have more than one chronic illness.

- A Canadian study of the medical records of 980 family practice patients found that 9 out of 10 patients had multiple chronic conditions. For patients ages 18 to 44, 68% of women and 72% of men had more than one illness at the same time. For patients 45 to 64, 95% of women and 89% of men had multiple medical conditions.

This prevalence of multimorbidity rose to an astonishing 99% of women and 97% of men age 65 and older. Among this oldest age group, 74% of the men and 77% of the women suffered from five or more chronic health problems at the same time! This study is highly credible because it examined actual medical records.

- In 2004, Americans with Medicare saw an average of seven different physicians in a year. Ninety-six percent of the money Medicare spent was to treat people with multiple chronic conditions.

- Medical doctors reviewing studies published worldwide concluded that multimorbidity afflicts 60% of people aged 55 to 74 and that half the patients with chronic illness have more than one.

You Pay In Every Way
In addition to the intense suffering of patients and their families, health care costs continue to soar to fund treatment of this staggering burden of disease. On average, a person with five or more chronic conditions incurs 15 times more medical costs in a year than does someone with no chronic conditions.

As a percent of the Gross Domestic Product (GDP), total health care costs in the U.S. rose from about 5% in 1960 to more than 16% in 2007. Researchers predict that by 2016, health care will eat up almost 20% of the GDP. People get sick regardless of the economy. So in a recession, health care will absorb an even greater slice of the GDP.

A federal study projects that by 2017, health care will cost government, businesses, and patients in the U.S. $4.3 trillion, doubling the amount spent in 2007. These rising costs make covering all citizens for health care an expensive goal, while families with health insurance are likely to be socked with much of the increased costs in higher premiums, deductibles, and copayments.

Think of the missed opportunities for using health care dollars to instead fund education, infrastructure, alternative energy, parks, environmental clean up, and other positive uses for money now being soaked up to treat chronic disease, which accounts for 83% of all health care spending. Or, taxes could simply be cut. *You pay the high financial cost of unchecked chronic illness through health insurance premiums, out-of-pocket expenses for medical care and drugs, and through your taxes.*

How Many Ways Can You Be Sick?

Here's a sample of the dizzying associations among specific medical conditions:

- Gum disease, known as gingivitis when mild and periodontal disease as it progresses, is seldom thought of as deadly. Yet if you have gum disease, you are significantly more likely to develop atherosclerosis (artery disease), diabetes, kidney disease, osteoporosis, Alzheimer's disease, stroke, and even cancer. If you're pregnant, you have a higher risk of preterm labor.
- If you suffer from depression, you're more likely than the average person to have or develop heart disease, rapid heart failure, allergies, and autoimmune disorders. Depressed adults are twice as likely to develop dementia when they get older and are also more prone to become diabetic and develop osteoporosis. Depressed pregnant women have twice the risk of delivering their baby prematurely.
- People with asthma have gastroesophageal reflux disease (GERD) more frequently than those without asthma.
- Patients with Barrett esophagus, a worrisome condition related to GERD, are more likely to have metabolic syndrome, a precursor of diabetes.
- People with metabolic syndrome are more likely to become schizophrenic.
- Adults with psoriasis are more likely to suffer a heart attack, stroke, coronary artery calcification, and joint problems.

Psoriasis sufferers are almost twice as likely to die from any cause than are people who don't have this skin condition.

- Men and women with migraine headaches have a higher chance than those without migraines of serious heart problems, heart attacks, and stroke.
- If you have rheumatoid arthritis, you're almost three times as likely to have heart disease as the general population. Rheumatoid arthritis and systemic lupus erythematosus increase the risk of death from a heart attack or stroke 50% more than the level of the general population.
- Having obstructive sleep apnea increases your risk for high blood pressure.
- Patients with restless legs syndrome are about twice as likely as others to have a stroke or heart disease; the risk goes up with more frequent and severe restless legs symptoms.

The discouraging list of associations among various chronic illnesses just keeps rolling on.

- Patients with inflammatory bowel disease (IBD), including Crohn's disease and ulcerative colitis, are more likely to have asthma, arthritis, bronchitis, psoriasis, pericarditis, and multiple sclerosis. Those with IBD have a 40% higher risk of a bone fracture of their spine, hip, wrist, or rib, regardless of whether they take steroids, and four to six times the risk of neuropathy or carpal tunnel syndrome. Women with IBD are twice as likely to have a low birth weight or premature baby.
- As many as 70% of those with fibromyalgia have the symptoms of chronic fatigue syndrome.
- Diabetes, hypertension, high cholesterol, and smoking all strongly raise the probability of developing dementia, not to mention cardiovascular disease. Diabetes also significantly raises the risk of hip fracture and pancreatic cancer.

- Clogged arteries raise the risk of hip fractures in women after menopause.
- Cardiovascular disease substantially increases your likelihood of chronic kidney disease.
- Developing early age-related macular degeneration puts you at about twice the risk of having a stroke.
- Sudden hearing loss ups your risk of having a stroke by about 50%.
- If you have Parkinson's disease, there's an increased chance you'll go on to develop Alzheimer's disease as well.
- Men with gout have a 30% greater risk of dying from cardiovascular disease than other men.
- Women who develop preeclampsia, a dangerous pregnancy-related condition, are five times as likely to develop high blood pressure and three times as likely to develop diabetes as women with uneventful pregnancies.
- Women with endometriosis were 62% more likely to develop melanoma than other women. Women with diabetes are 70% more likely to develop endometrial cancer.
- A study of women with an average age of 80 found those who had a premature baby decades earlier had about three times the risk for cardiovascular disease when elderly. This association held even though the births had been, on average, 57 years earlier!

Think about these results for a minute. The rest of your life is at stake.

If you're already sick, how does this list of findings make you feel? Do you fear you are doomed to a lifetime of high medical costs, reliance on family and friends for help, long waits in doctor's offices, being poked, X-rayed, and cut open, cruising the aisles of your local drugstore for over-the-counter remedies while your multiple prescriptions are readied?

Take heart! You can pursue a simple way out of this medical maze and back into the world of health. This opportunity may slip by unless you make some uncomplicated changes in your food choices.

Is It All One Illness?

Authors of studies reporting that one chronic illness so often leads to another are usually puzzled by their own findings. Sometimes the researchers advance a couple of theories or ideas, but the bottom line is that no one so far has put forward an accepted explanation.

Yet all the dots are there to connect and understand chronic disease. *In fact, the key to comprehending, preventing, and reversing chronic illnesses may lie in their interrelationships. Read on for a fresh way of looking at why you get sick and what actions may pave the way to wellness.*

Think about the last time you had the flu. Multiple symptoms resulted in feeling wretched. For example, you might have had respiratory symptoms—stuffed nose, sinus problems, cough, and clogged lungs. You likely had a fever, overwhelming fatigue and weakness, chills, headache, and aching joints. You probably lost your appetite and might have been nauseous with intestinal issues.

Did you label each of these symptoms as a different illness? No, you understood you had the flu, and that the diverse problems in so many systems of your body manifested infection from one virus. You might have caught the same bug as a family member or co-worker, yet each of you had somewhat different symptoms with varying recovery paths.

Consider the idea that chronic illnesses are similar to the flu, with what appear to be different diseases really just diverse aspects of one root cause. For the flu, the origin of all your symptoms is infection by a powerful virus. For most chronic disease, symptoms may originate in chronic inflammation, sometimes local but more often systemic throughout your body. While this is a new idea, it does explain many observations and research findings, and so deserves attention and study.

Two European physicians, writing in the prestigious journal *Lancet,* advocated for this idea as it relates to chronic obstructive pulmonary disease (COPD). These insightful researchers proposed the term "chronic systemic inflammatory syndrome" to explain why COPD is seldom an isolated diagnosis. Patients with COPD are 50% to 80% more likely to develop diabetes and are also prone to skeletal muscle abnormalities, high blood pressure, cardiovascular disease, heart failure, ulcers, osteoporosis, and cancer. For these patients, body-wide inflammation is mainly the result of years of cigarette smoking.

When you understand that inflammation may be a root cause of most chronic illness, you can appreciate why having any one of these diseases so often leads to another. Each disease can appear to be different, but in fact they may be grouped together just like the symptoms of the flu.

The Story Condensed

Just as drunk driving increases the chances you will get into an accident, risk factors increase the likelihood that you will miss out on the health you want.

If you have one chronic illness, your chances of developing another one skyrocket. Research suggests most chronic illness is strongly related to chronic inflammation, which helps explain why people with one diagnosis so often suffer from others. "It's all one illness" is a fresh way of looking at chronic illness, and research in this direction might uncover startling results.

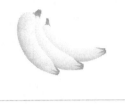

CHAPTER 13

Perfect Defenses

Theories of illness change over time, and today's accepted wisdom was yesterday's heresy. Think about how doctors once ridiculed the germ theory of disease and, even in the 20th century, gave out cigarettes to their patients to reduce stress.

The focus on inflammation is a quantum shift in how modern scientists think about health and disease. Medical journals are filled with tens of thousands of articles documenting the fact that inflammation is a critical factor in many chronic illnesses, such as cardiovascular disease, diabetes, and arthritis, which are epidemic in developed countries.

The more you know about inflammation, the better you'll understand why you are sick and how you can enjoy Perfect Health. As you read on, you'll understand how the Perfect Formula Diet might play a key role in maintaining the optimal balance between pro- and anti-inflammatory forces in your body. First, here are some basic facts.

Inflammation: Standing Between You And Death
Inflammation is a set of orchestrated steps your body initiates when threatened by any potentially harmful external or internal factor that could injure your cells or interfere with healthy functioning.

This is a critical survival mechanism shared by all creatures with blood circulation. Hundreds of different biological and chemical dynamics interrelate in the inflammatory process. Your immune and nervous systems are the most critical players in inflammation.

Think of inflammation as the "first responder" when the health or survival of your body's cells or tissues are at risk. Police and fire department first responders need look-outs for danger, messengers and communication systems to spread the alarm, and multiple weapons and defensive and recovery strategies to cope with challenges that might range from fire and bombs to bank robbers and train wrecks.

Inflammation also has all these components: the look-outs, alarm systems, and numerous offensive, defensive, and recovery components. At the cellular level, sentries scan for danger, effective pathways spread the word when a threat is recognized, and both offensive and defensive components deploy as necessary to make sure you survive danger and heal afterward.

Inflammation is more than a first responder and has a vital part in healing and the return to optimal functioning after the threat is defeated. So inflammation has roles similar to both a fire crew, putting out the flames, and the construction workers who come in afterward to repair the damage.

Provoking Inflammation

The components of the inflammatory process are always on the lookout to defend you, guard your health, and ensure your survival. This book uses the word "inflammators" for the perils that activate inflammation. This word, although not medical jargon, clearly conveys the effect of these potential menaces to your survival.

Your body is designed to detect and respond quickly and decisively to a wide range of inflammators:

- Harmful bacteria, viruses, and parasites which may infect you
- Injuries and burns
- Excess heat or cold

- Oxygen deprivation
- Smoking
- Too much or not enough food and nutrients
- Excess cholesterol
- Insect bites
- Splinters
- Chronic irritation that damages cells (for example, from something rubbing against your skin)
- Radiation
- Products of your body's own metabolism, such as free radicals
- Toxic chemicals in your food, water, air, personal care and cleaning products, and living environment
- Proteins that are different from yours (for example, from a transplanted organ, blood transfusion, or animal foods)
- Malignant cells
- Your own nonmalignant cells, if they are damaged or cannot properly function as your body needs them to

Inflammation's Power

The inflammatory process uses many strategies, both offensive and defensive, to counter threats to your health and survival.

The first step of the inflammatory process attacks the inflammator with the goal of containing and destroying it. Physicians thousands of years ago recognized the classic signs of early inflammation: heat, swelling, pain, and redness. Different aspects of the inflammatory process wall off the inflammator, dilute it with fluids (thus the swelling), mark it for destruction by the body's protective cells, and attack or engulf it.

During this part of the process you may run a fever, which often helps your body gain an upper hand on infections, as some microbes have a tough time surviving the higher temperature. You're also likely to experience fatigue, lethargy, reduced appetite, aching joints and muscles, and pain as the inflammatory process launches a strong strike.

In fact, you may become hypersensitive to pain in parts of your body that aren't the center of inflammation. This is because substances your body releases during the inflammatory process increase the sensitivity of nerves to pain.

These symptoms have a survival advantage, for example, by conserving your energy to fight the inflammator and keeping you from injuring the affected body part even more by touching or moving it. Your symptoms are telling you something and you are well advised to listen. On the other hand, if the inflammator is only a mild threat and the resulting inflammatory response is localized and over quickly, you might not experience any symptoms.

Once the inflammator is deactivated, the inflammatory response moves on to promote healing and recovery by stimulating cell and blood vessel growth. Your injured cells may recover or new cells or scar tissue may form.

You can see that, although long-term inflammation is strongly related to chronic illness, the optimal solution is *not* to deactivate or even weaken your inflammatory response. Without the ability to respond to and heal from danger, your body is defenseless and your life could be quite short.

Measuring Inflammation: Knowing Where You Stand

C-reactive protein (CRP) and interleukin-6 (IL-6) are two substances your body produces early in the inflammatory process. Both play a role in protection from inflammators. One action of CRP is to bind to invading microbes in order to mark them for recognition by other cells that will destroy and dispose of these threats. Think of CRP as shouting: "Look, danger over here, help." CRP also helps get rid of dead cells.

IL-6 has multiple functions, including inducing fever, activating immune cells, and stimulating your body to make healing and anti-inflammatory proteins. IL-6 enhances the synthesis of CRP.

Scientists most often use both CRP and IL-6 as nonspecific markers of inflammation, indicating the level of inflammation but not what caused it. Both these measures are useful, but also crude. The amount of inflammation you experience is a balance of pro- and anti-inflammatory forces. So you can be in an inflammatory state if anti-inflammatory substances are low, not just if pro-inflammatory substances are elevated.

Moreover, there are hundreds of substances involved in the inflammatory process, so isolating one or two provides only limited insight as to the exact condition of your body. Nonetheless, both CRP and IL-6 are useful in indicating the amount of inflammation present in your body and many of the studies discussed in this book use them.

The Coin Has Another Side

The cycle of inflammation that recognizes and responds to an inflammator, destroys or inactivates it, and makes sure your body returns to normal function is called acute inflammation. While the experience of acute inflammation is not enjoyable, it's also relatively short-lived and is critical to survival. The acute phase of inflammation may last a few days to a few weeks.

For chronic illness, one key underlying cause is often chronic, as opposed to acute inflammation. Chronic inflammation is prolonged and poses a different dynamic than acute inflammation. While acute inflammation is protective, chronic inflammation is damaging.

Excessive or prolonged inflammation is like friendly fire on the battlefield—potentially just as dangerous as any enemy. For example, sepsis, a treatment-resistant condition that ends in multiple organ failure and often death, occurs when your body's inflammatory response to infection gets out of control.

During chronic inflammation, attacks on a current inflammator and healing from past inflammators are happening at the same time. Since each of these processes was designed to work best as a separate phase, neither process operates as well as it might. You become susceptible to internal and external threats and tissue healing doesn't proceed as it should.

When inflammation results from a single challenge, even if that exposure is major, the inflammation tends to be time-limited. When an inflammator menaces you repeatedly or for a long period of time, inflammation is more likely to be chronic and self-perpetuating. This is because ongoing inflammation produces toxic substances which themselves trigger additional inflammation.

The fact that your Perfect Body falls into this unnatural state has much to do with your food choices and chemicals in your environment. As your read on, the big picture and the healing role of the Perfect Formula Diet will become clear.

Balance Is Everything

Inflammation may become chronic either because a powerful inflammator is still present or because the mechanisms that end acute inflammation fail. Normally, acute inflammation resolves because your body produces large quantities of anti-inflammatory substances after the pro-inflammatory substances have done their work. *The pro-inflammatory substances themselves are one trigger for the production of the anti-inflammatory molecules, once acute inflammation has done its job.*

Your health hinges on the balance of pro- and anti-inflammatory forces. When anti-inflammatory forces predominate, your body cannot defend itself strongly from internal and external threats. When a pro-inflammatory dynamic has the upper hand, inflammation outstays its useful function and becomes chronic, damaging your body's tissues in the process.

You can think of this as similar to driving. The brakes (anti-inflammatory forces) are just as important as the accelerator (pro-inflammatory forces) to keep you cruising at a safe speed that gets you where you want to go.

However, separating pro- and anti-inflammatory processes is tricky. Think about a thermostat. When a room is too cold, the thermostat sends a signal to the furnace to turn on the heat. You want the room to be warmer, but you don't want your furnace to blast unchecked. Once the room reaches the temperature you want, the thermostat sends another signal and the furnace shuts off. What turns off the thermostat? The warmth of its previous operation, of course.

In the same way that heat turns off a furnace when the thermostat senses enough is enough, pro-inflammatory substances trigger the release of anti-inflammatory substances to keep the level of inflammation under control. Your nervous system and hormones also play important roles in keeping inflammation at the optimal level.

So, paradoxically, suppressing inflammation through ill-timed interventions (such as certain medications) may actually keep the anti-inflammatory process from properly launching. Chronic inflammation can be one result.

When the inflammatory process is out of balance and the timing of switching from attack to healing mode is skewed, your body can be susceptible to both inadequate inflammation and excessive inflammation.

Simplistically tinkering with your body is likely to do more harm than good. The rebound effect is one example of this. Rebound can occur when you have been suppressing the inflammatory response with medication. In order to maintain balance, your body must cut back on its own production of anti-inflammatory substances. This ensures that the inflammatory response does not get too muted to respond to microbes or other threats.

When the anti-inflammatory medication is halted, excessive inflammation may rebound until the body has time to ramp up production again of its own anti-inflammatory substances. To illustrate this, scientists have found that withdrawing aspirin (an anti-inflammatory medication) in people who have been taking it regularly significantly increases the risk of heart attack and stroke (which may be end-points of an inflammatory process).

In a healthy environment and with Perfect Foods, your body is best able to maintain the ideal balance of pro- and anti-inflammatory forces. The intricate mechanisms built in to do this are far superior to external interventions, which do not fully account for the complexity of the process.

Immunity: Your "First Responder" Powerhouse

If inflammation is a "first responder," then your immune system is the strongest force it deploys. Your immune system, a highly organized network of about three trillion specialized cells and tissues throughout your body, is your most powerful agent for destroying dangerous inflammators. Even if only one component of this intricate network is missing or not working properly, the entire system can malfunction.

Your immune system's actions are the basis for most of the inflammatory process. The immune system is central to the inflammatory process the same way the police are the basis for the response to a bank robbery.

Some immune system cells react to any inflammator, while others have a specific job and may be called in only occasionally. Think of police officers who are trained for any emergency vs. units such as SWAT teams, gang units, undercover operations, bomb squads, and so on which operate only in special circumstances. The specialized parts of the immune system have memory and can learn from prior contact with certain inflammators.

Your nervous, hormonal, and immune systems interact in important ways. For example, your nervous system helps monitor and adjust the strength of immune system response so it's optimal. Immune system cells can make nerves more sensitive to pain. Some hormones can dampen immune system activity to make sure it doesn't become stronger or more widespread than necessary.

Catalogue Of Misery

If you live in a developed country, chances are high that you'll die from chronic inflammation contributing to one of a long list of diagnoses. Disability and pain from chronic inflammation will likely haunt you along the way.

Scientists have demonstrated that numerous chronic illnesses are strongly tied to chronic inflammation. Here are some examples:

- Cardiovascular disease in its many forms: high blood pressure, heart attack, chronic heart failure, peripheral artery disease, stroke
- Type 2 diabetes and metabolic syndrome
- Autoimmune disorders, including rheumatoid arthritis, lupus, multiple sclerosis, type 1 diabetes
- Depression, autism, cognitive decline, and Alzheimer's disease
- Asthma
- Chronic obstructive pulmonary disease (COPD)
- Sinusitis and chronic bronchitis
- Allergies
- Psoriasis
- Age-related macular degeneration and cataracts
- Inflammatory bowel disease
- Barrett esophagus
- Gum disease
- Sleep apnea
- Osteoporosis
- Osteoarthritis and other chronic pain, including headaches, fibromyalgia, chronic fatigue syndrome, and low back pain
- Premature birth
- Cancer

As studies of multimorbidity show, these diagnoses are interlinked. Researchers would do well to investigate how the whole lot may be a diverse manifestation of a chronic inflammatory syndrome.

Inflamm-Aging

In fact, chronic inflammation may accelerate aging because, after decades of fighting inflammators, your body is more susceptible to pro-inflammatory mechanisms and has a harder time maintaining balance. Scientists have labeled this chronic, low-level inflammatory state "inflamm-aging."

The diagnoses that manifest chronic inflammation *are* those that, way too often, define aging in developed countries: arthritis, heart disease, brittle bones, Alzheimer's disease, stroke, macular degeneration, cataracts, chronic pain, and cancer.

Frailty, another hallmark of inflamm-aging, is recognized by diffuse symptoms and progressive loss of strength. Older people with high levels of inflammatory markers are at greater risk of disability and have higher death rates.

Centenarians—those 100 years old or more—in good health often have a genetic boost that helps them keep a favorable balance of pro- and anti-inflammatory processes. *Even without such lucky genetics, you can mimic this balance into your older years through Perfect Foods and other everyday choices.*

The Smoking Gun

Here's another critical fact. The smoking gun connecting chronic inflammation to chronic illness is the level of inflammatory markers in sick vs. healthy people. Researchers most often use CRP and IL-6 to measure inflammation, as described earlier. Here is a tiny sampling of thousands of studies all pointing in the same direction.

- Aging: older people with higher levels of IL-6 tend to experience greater disability, more chronic illness, and increased death rates, while those with higher amounts of IL-6 and/or CRP tend to have weaker muscles and poor physical abilities.
- Cardiovascular disease: the weight of evidence connecting increased indicators of systemic inflammation to heart and blood vessel disease is overwhelming and widely recognized in the medical community. For example, women with high CRP are twice as likely to have a heart attack or stroke than are women with only high cholesterol, and men exhibit a similar pattern. Women with the highest levels of CRP and

IL-6 are 10 times as likely to die from a heart attack as are women with the lowest levels of these inflammatory markers.

- Hypertension: if you have elevated CRP, you are more likely to have high blood pressure, even without other risk factors for this condition.
- Diabetes: patients with type 2 diabetes have higher CRP levels, while those with elevated inflammatory markers were more likely to develop type 2 diabetes if they didn't already have it. Type 1 diabetes is also associated with increased systemic inflammatory markers.

Scientists have discovered more.

- Depression: patients with depression have, on average, significantly higher levels of CRP, IL-6, and other inflammatory markers than do people who are not depressed.
- Arthritis: patients with either osteoarthritis or rheumatoid arthritis are likely to have elevated levels of IL-6 and other markers of inflammation.
- Cognitive decline: if you have a higher level of CRP, you're prone to perform worse on tests of memory, attention, speed of perception and reaction, and mental flexibility.
- Alzheimer's disease: a study that followed men for 28 years found that those with the highest CRP levels at the beginning of the study had four to five times the rate of Alzheimer's at the end of the study.
- Psoriasis: patients with psoriasis are likely to have significantly higher levels of CRP than study participants who do not have this condition.
- Cancer: if you have increased levels of CRP, you are twice as likely to develop colon cancer and are less likely to survive after treatment for several cancer types.
- Preterm delivery: pregnant women with higher CRP levels have an increased risk of delivering their baby too early.

Researchers can also look at amounts of anti-inflammatory markers. Patients with chronic pain throughout their bodies had low levels of anti-inflammatory substances.

Studies of anti-inflammatory over-the-counter drugs, such as aspirin and nonsteroidal anti-inflammatory drugs (NSAIDs), indicate that countering inflammation may reduce the risk of some chronic inflammatory illnesses. *Note these drugs may have serious side effects and are not beneficial for everyone. Don't use these drugs without an approval from your doctor. Also keep the dangerous rebound effect in mind if you do take any of these drugs and then stop.*

- Long-term use of aspirin or NSAIDs may reduce the risk of certain cancers, including colon, lung, esophagus, breast, prostate, skin, and stomach cancers.
- Diabetics who take aspirin may have reduced symptoms of their illness.
- Taking NSAIDs over a five year period may reduce the risk of developing Alzheimer's disease.
- Low doses of aspirin may lower the risk of dying from cardiovascular disease.

Have you known or read about people who appeared to be fit and not any sicker than most of their peers, and then unexpectedly died from a heart attack or were stricken with cancer? In general, if your CRP is elevated, you're at increased risk for poor outcomes from chronic illness and have a higher risk of death even if you seem to be healthy.

Inflammatory Burden

Think of your inflammatory burden as the weight of all the inflammators that activate your inflammatory defensive response. The greater your inflammatory burden, the more pro-inflammatory substances are needed to fight threats and the more anti-inflammatory substances your body must produce to keep the resulting inflammation under control.

With these two opposing forces—pro- and anti-inflammatory—coursing strongly through your body, there may be significant room for dangerous under- or over-reactions, not to mention exhaustion of one or more of your body's systems. This is not a stable, balanced situation.

Again, the analogy of a thermostat can enhance understanding. Think of a room with closed windows and tight weather stripping on a windy winter day. The thermostat will need to turn on the furnace on occasion to keep the room at a comfortable temperature. However, there will be few drafts and the temperature should not vary more than a few degrees from the ideal, assuming your home systems are working properly.

Now, think of the same room, but with open windows blasted by wintry gusts. The thermostat will be permanently on. The room temperature can swing wildly, depending on how strongly the wind blew recently and whether the air in the furnace had time to properly warm before being powered through the vent. You're not likely to be very comfortable in this room.

The situation with the adequate weather stripping is like your body with a low inflammatory burden. With few inflammators "blowing through," your inflammatory processes are more likely to remain low key and countervailing anti-inflammatory processes can operate at a similarly reduced level. You can enjoy balance and stable health.

The open windows scenario portrays your body under a heavy inflammatory burden. You're constantly beset with powerful threats that trigger inflammation. Equally strong anti-inflammatory processes must be launched to keep inflammation in check. Staying in balance is tricky, and pockets of heat and cold (excessive and inadequate inflammation) are likely.

Your body, like the furnace with no down time, gets worn out before its time. Even anti-inflammatory drugs do little to mitigate this situation in the long run. In practice, this analogy corresponds to the scientific findings that, in chronic inflammation, both pro- and anti-inflammatory substances are increased two- to four-fold over normal levels and the risk of many chronic illnesses skyrockets.

The takeaway lesson is to avoid unnecessary inflammators. This strategy conserves your energy for menaces that cannot be sidestepped and maximizes your ability to keep a low, healthy balance of pro- and anti-inflammatory forces.

The Story Condensed

Inflammation is your "first responder" that protects against a long list of hazards that could injure or kill you ("inflammators") and is also an integral part of the healing process after injury. Inflammators include microbes, injury, toxic chemicals, malignant cells, and foreign proteins (such as those from animal foods). C-reactive protein (CRP) and interleukin-6 (IL-6) are important markers of inflammation.

While acute inflammation is protective, chronic inflammation is damaging. When an inflammator menaces you repeatedly or for a long period of time, or when the anti-inflammatory process is stalled, inflammation is more likely to be chronic and self-perpetuating.

Your health is strongly linked to the balance of pro- and anti-inflammatory forces. When anti-inflammatory forces predominate, your body cannot defend itself strongly from internal and external threats. When a pro-inflammatory dynamic has the upper hand, inflammation outstays its useful function and becomes chronic, damaging your body's tissues in the process.

In a healthy environment and with Perfect Foods, your body is best able to exquisitely maintain the ideal balance of pro- and anti-inflammatory forces. The intricate mechanisms built in to do this are far superior to external interventions, which do not fully account for the complexity of the process.

If you live in a developed country, chances are high that you will die from chronic inflammation contributing to one of a long list of diagnoses. Disability and pain from chronic inflammation will likely haunt you along the way. Chronic illnesses strongly linked to inflammation include cardiovascular disease, diabetes, cancer, stroke, Alzheimer's, arthritis, migraine headaches, and many others. Aging itself is linked to chronic inflammation.

You are well advised to minimize your inflammatory burden by avoiding inflammators whenever you can. The Perfect Formula Diet is the surest way to avoid most everyday inflammators in your life, as the rest of this book demonstrates.

CHAPTER 14

Perfect Balance

You may be wondering how chronic inflammation affects your health so profoundly. Diverse mechanisms for this harm, which research indicates may be related to your food choices, may trigger malfunction in multiple body systems.

- Inflamed blood vessels cause a no-cell-left-untouched traffic jam in your body, preventing delivery of adequate oxygen and nutrients. This process weakens every bodily system and predisposes you to form dangerous blood clots that may result in heart attack or stroke.
- Some foreign proteins (especially those in animal foods) can closely match your own proteins, confusing the inflammatory process into attacking your tissues in an autoimmune process. With this barrage of inflammators, your immune system can become hair trigger responsive, resulting in an increased susceptibility to allergies and asthma.
- Large combinations of bonded cells, composed of inflammators and your body's defensive immune cells, are like splinters in your joints and other tissues.
- Pro-inflammatory messenger substances in your body make your nerves hypersensitive to pain, and even undamaged

nerves may begin sending pain signals when you're in a chronic inflammatory state.

• Your HDL cholesterol, usually viewed as a heart attack preventive, can alter its functioning and become pro-inflammatory regardless of its level; this happens because how a specific substance functions in your body depends on the overall chemistry of your body, which changes in chronic inflammation.

This chapter and the next describe these contributors to illness and the Perfect Formula Diet road to trimness and health. As you can see, no single factor is sufficiently powerful to explain all illness. While these chapters describe critical dynamics of disease, scientists will have much to discover.

Plaque: Your 70,000–Mile Traffic Jam

A typical adult has about 70,000 miles of blood vessels delivering nutrients, oxygen, and other vital necessities. This awesome living highway carries the essentials of life to each cell and carts away the toxic wastes that normal metabolism generates. The exchange between your blood and each cell occurs in the tiniest blood vessels called capillaries.

When your blood flows freely and unimpeded, every cell can function optimally. When your blood vessels become clogged, however, cells starve for nutrients and oxygen, while wastes at the cellular level cannot be adequately eliminated. All 100 trillion cells in your body suffer and general physical malfunctioning can result.

Chronic inflammation is one driving force in the progressive growth of plaque inside your blood vessels. Plaque, a substance that chokes blood flow to create a 70,000-mile traffic jam, consists of a protein coating over a core of fats and dead cells that the inflammatory process produces.

Plaque: The Road Block Grows

Plaque is not a passive deposit on your blood vessel walls. Instead, it's the end result of a chronic inflammatory process that progresses over a long period of time (beginning in childhood in developed countries). Your diet plays a major role in controlling this inflammatory process.

Plaque formation begins when the inner surface of your blood vessel wall is irritated or damaged by excess cholesterol, metabolic waste products, infection, or some other inflammator. Just as any other injury would do, this threat to your blood vessel triggers an inflammatory response geared to contain and repair the damage.

Through a chronic, multi-step inflammatory process, your blood vessel wall becomes thicker and lined with plaque deposits. Your doctor may refer to this process as atherosclerosis, hardening of the arteries, or cardiovascular disease.

Heart attacks and strokes occur when the plaque coating ruptures, generating a blood clot that can block all blood flow to part of your heart or brain. Chronic inflammation also destabilizes plaque, making it more likely that the coating will tear and release the dangerous core.

Newly formed, unstable plaque with a soft coating is most likely to rupture, while older plaque, with its tough cover, is likely to retain its form and not generate a life-threatening blood clot. Medical treatment that opens a stretch of blocked arteries using stents, by-pass surgery, or some other mechanical means doesn't solve the problem. The 70,000-mile traffic jam remains (with one short open stretch of road) and the patches of soft unpredictable plaque elsewhere in your body remain poised to rupture.

After eating a high fat/high calorie meal with animal foods and manufactured foods, your blood vessels tend to shut down even more until your body can clear the fat that inundates your blood vessels. Your blood will look cloudy, perhaps even white, from all the fat in it. Clumps of fat and red blood cells stop your cells from getting even the reduced amount of oxygen they usually must make do with. Eating small amounts of Perfect Foods as "side orders" does little or nothing to stop this effect.

Sometimes calcium is deposited in plaque, which makes blood vessel walls brittle and stiff. These unnaturally rigid blood vessels don't function properly and are susceptible to tears that lead to internal bleeding. Conversely, the inflamed, weakened artery walls can develop dangerous bulges called aneurysms.

Still another unpleasant possibility is that plaque becomes infected. Bacteria can grow in an injured artery wall, causing still more inflammation and damage to your blood vessels. However, healthy artery walls keep bacteria at bay.

Mistaken Identity

If clogged, damaged blood vessels weren't enough, chronic inflammation contributes to more harm. Your inflammatory response, spearheaded by your immune system, has the challenging task of guarding you from millions of potential inflammators, many of which cannot be predicted or known in advance. At the same time, your immune system must refrain from attacking beneficial and necessary proteins and other substances.

The goal of the immune system is sometimes described as distinguishing between "self" and "non-self" but it's actually far trickier than this. Some of your "self," such as malignant cells or badly damaged cells that can no longer do their jobs, are threats that are properly destroyed by a healthy immune system. Some foreign proteins, such as those of beneficial (probiotic) bacteria, are fundamental to survival and must be allowed to thrive. Many other foreign proteins, such as pollen in the air, are neither harmful nor helpful; you do best when your immune system ignores these.

If your body attacked every "non-self" protein it encountered, you would die from massive inflammation very quickly. Conversely, if every "self" protein were left alone, malignancy would thrive from your earliest days. Your immune system accomplishes a marvelous balancing act every moment through pattern recognition receptors.

The more foreign proteins your immune system must deal with and the more these proteins are similar to your own, the harder it becomes for your immune system to distinguish among invaders that should be attacked, harmless substances in the environment, and your own healthy cells. Your immune system becomes both fatigued and hypersensitive.

Molecular mimicry is a process sparked by foreign proteins that have amino acid sequences (one portion of the entire amino acid chain) very similar or identical to those of some of your own proteins. Your body makes defensive cells to attack the invaders, and these defenses can then turn on the similar "self" cells.

For example, one amino acid sequence in a dairy protein is quite similar to that in the collagen in your joints. Your body may manufacture defenses against the proteins in cow's milk because these are foreign proteins and perceived as a potential threats. These same defenses may end up attacking your own joint tissues, resulting in rheumatoid arthritis. Proteins in cow's milk have also been closely linked to the development of type 1 diabetes as certain specific dairy proteins are look-alikes for pancreatic cells.

You can think of this as a case of mistaken identity contributing to autoimmune diseases such as type 1 diabetes, rheumatoid arthritis, lupus, myasthenia gravis, Graves disease, multiple sclerosis, ulcerative colitis, and psoriatic arthritis. Other causative factors for autoimmune diseases include certain infections, chemicals, and drugs, especially if these over-stimulate your immune system or damage your cells.

For some common autoimmune diseases, an identical twin of a patient with such an illness may have only a 15% to 30% chance of developing the same condition. This fact shows that genetics is not destiny for autoimmune disorders.

Nature Should Make You Well, Not Sick

The hypersensitive state that may occur in chronic inflammation can also aggravate allergic reactions to food or environmental substances that would be best ignored. In these cases, the hair-trigger inflammatory response is itself the problem.

The inability to tolerate pollen, for example, would lead to a lower probability of survival in nature, which is where humans have lived for most of our history. Why would a condition such as hay fever, which has negative survival advantage, develop? Scientists should investigate the role of chronic inflammation in causing the immune system to react strongly to harmless proteins, such as those in plant pollens.

Here's an important health fact. Across most areas of the world, especially in developed countries, the incidence of many allergies, asthma, and immune system disorders has increased by a factor of two to four. Researchers have many theories about this skyrocketing prevalence, but none is generally accepted.

Keep reading for some fresh ideas about the root of chronic inflammation contributing to much of this increase. These ideas definitely require additional research, but are promising based on studies already done.

Splinters You Can't Get Out

One of the strategies your body uses to neutralize an inflammator is to send an immune system cell to bind with, destroy, or engulf it. The resulting combination of your own immune cell bonded to the original inflammator may be large enough to settle out of your body's fluids and into tissue. When this happens, the combination acts like a splinter, causing its own irritation and inflammation.

If these bonded pairs are forming more quickly than you can dispose of them, they may settle into blood vessel walls, or into your kidneys, joints, eyes, or other tissues. This result is more likely during chronic inflammation when combinations form constantly. Damage and pain, including arthritis, may be the result.

Food: Chronic Inflammation's Patron Or Enemy

Okay, you may be thinking, this information is all very interesting, but what is it doing in this book? What does it have to do with Perfect Foods and the Perfect Formula Diet? The answer is—*chronic inflammation is strongly affected by what you eat.*

Animals cannot make their own nourishment through photosynthesis, and must consume plants or other animals to get what they need to live. So your immune system needs to defend you against invaders from the animal kingdom, such as bacteria, viruses, and parasites, which may be looking at you as their next meal.

Since these potential enemies can morph into new forms very quickly, your immune system needs to be able to identify animal protein *patterns* and not just a specific fixed list of microbes and parasites. Your immune system is on the lookout for *foreign animal proteins*—that is, any animal proteins other than your own.

Your immune system is *not* generally watching for plant proteins, because plants are not going to infect you. Plants happily thrive in the soil under the sun and rain, and have no need for your cells or organ systems to supply their need for food or reproduction. There's little reason for plant proteins to activate a healthy human immune system (but they may provoke an allergic reaction from a damaged or susceptible immune system).

The only exception would be a fungus, because these plants lack chlorophyll and so must rely on other organisms for food, just as animals do. Fungus infections in humans range from dangerous to cosmetically annoying, so your immune system also needs to be able to recognize and defend against these potential threats.

The Perfect Formula Diet works to strengthen your immune system while balancing pro-and anti-inflammatory forces in your body. This eating plan spares you from the animal proteins that may aggravate chronic inflammation when you eat them on a regular basis.

Eating Your Way To Chronic Inflammation

Scientists are just beginning to document the effect of diet on chronic inflammation. Some studies indicate that certain foreign proteins—possibly animal proteins in food—tend to raise CRP levels, while Perfect Foods lower CRP levels. Inflammation, in turn, increases "leaky gut" so more foreign proteins can cross from your digestive system into your blood. In this dangerous dynamic, foreign proteins may provoke inflammation, which would then inflame your intestines and allow still more unwanted proteins to enter your body.

European scientists analyzed 108 studies, concluding that manufactured foods and trans-fatty acids aggravate inflammation throughout the body, while fruit, vegetables, nuts, whole grains, and omega-3 fatty acids are inflammation fighters. Additional results, which need to be bolstered by further research, strongly indicate that chronic inflammation is closely related to your food choices.

- A study of diabetic patients found that the group that ate less protein had significantly reduced CRP levels.
- In a study of 26 volunteers, one group followed a diet based 70% on complex carbohydrates, while another group chose a high protein (from animal foods) diet. Those on the lower protein diet enjoyed a drop in their CRP levels and an improvement in artery health. Those in the high protein group saw a 61% increase in CRP levels.
- Similar research with 32 overweight women found that, within a week of starting a diet based on animal foods, the women's CRP levels rose 25%. In contrast, women who got 60% of their energy from carbohydrates benefited from a 43% decrease in CRP.
- Two studies with rheumatoid arthritis patients on a 100% plant-based diet saw CRP levels decrease; researchers concluded that the animal-free diet protected the patients' arteries and was anti-inflammatory.
- People on a 100% plant-based raw foods diet had significantly lower levels of CRP than those of a similar age, sex, and economic status who ate a typical American diet.
- Couch potato adults on a plant-based diet had lower CRP levels than similarly inactive people eating a typical American diet.

- Eating Perfect Foods—fruits, vegetables, whole grains—lowers your CRP levels, indicating reduced chronic inflammation.
- Diets rich in fiber are associated with reduced CRP levels. Keep in mind that fiber is an indicator of Perfect Foods, because only these foods have high fiber levels. Animal foods contain no fiber, and most manufactured foods are depleted of the fiber in the whole plant.

A series of studies of the Pritikin Diet also indicates that eating a diet based on Perfect Foods with little or no animal foods can dramatically reduce chronic inflammation. This eating plan emphasizes nicely seasoned Perfect Foods and includes animal foods as an infrequent option in small amounts only.

- Twenty postmenopausal women on this diet saw their CRP fall by 45% in two weeks.
- Thirty-one obese men following this eating plan benefited from a 40% reduction in CRP in just three weeks.
- More than 100 medical journals have published studies showing beneficial health impact, permanent weight loss, and reduced CRP levels from the Pritikin Diet.

More Foreign Protein Hazards
Foreign proteins can contribute to inflammatory chronic illness however they get into the body, through diet or otherwise.

- Many slaughterhouse workers who inhaled microscopic particles of pigs' brains suffered an inflammatory autoimmune reaction with symptoms including pain, numbness, tingling, fatigue, and weakness. Scientists should intensively research whether the dietary animal proteins that encounter your immune system can excite similar autoimmune and inflammatory processes.

- Receiving a blood transfusion significantly raises the risk of developing an infection or having a heart attack, stroke, kidney problem, or other complication after surgery. Transfusion recipients were substantially more likely to die in the year after surgery, compared to similar patients who didn't get a transfusion. This potentially indicates harmful effects from the systemic inflammation that would follow an infusion of someone else's blood proteins into your body.

Anti- And Pro- Are Not The Ideals

The tremendous range and volume of inflammators in modern life—proteins in overabundant animal foods, chemicals in food, air, water, and cleaning and personal care products, radiation from our electronic gadgets, novel microbes, and other challenges—may put many citizens into a chronic inflammatory state that's a key factor in chronic illness. So you might think the best way to counter this condition is with massive anti-inflammatory drugs to beat the inflammation back down.

In fact, that would be a mistake. Going from a pro- to an anti-inflammatory extreme is not your goal. *Suppressing inflammation can be every bit as deadly as magnifying and prolonging inflammation. What you want is a balance of pro- and anti-inflammatory forces in your body. You want your immune system to be powerful without being hyperactive or hair trigger sensitive.*

If you just want to counter inflammation without getting to the root cause, then anti-inflammatory drugs may be your choice. *If you want to enhance your immune system without either provoking or suppressing it, then follow the Perfect Formula Diet.*

Perfect Foods help normalize the working of your immune system, so you can crush inflammators without overshooting the mark into a chronic inflammatory state. On the Perfect Formula Diet, you avoid any inflammators in animal and manufactured foods, so you're not constantly provoking an inflammatory response and setting the stage for chronic inflammation. The beneficial phytochemicals in Perfect

Foods strengthen your immune system so it can better knock out the inflammators you can't avoid.

The Perfect Formula Diet has a dual role in achieving balance. You drastically reduce both the everyday inflammators from food— thus lowering your inflammatory burden—and you strengthen your defensive forces so menaces to your health are overcome more quickly.

The role of Perfect Foods in achieving optimal health explains why your health can soar when you follow the Perfect Formula Diet, even if you are already at your Perfect Weight. As later chapters explain, also aim to minimize other inflammators so your immune system doesn't get exhausted, confused, and weakened.

The Story Condensed

Chronic inflammation can harm you and contribute to chronic illness in many ways. Starting in childhood in most developed countries, plaque clogs your blood vessels as the result of chronic inflammation, causing a 70,000-mile traffic jam that damages cells throughout your body. In addition:

- Some foreign proteins in food can closely match your own proteins, confusing the inflammatory process into attacking your own tissues in an autoimmune process.
- Large complexes, composed of inflammators and your body's defensive immune cells, are like painful splinters in your joints and other tissues.

Your immune system is on the lookout for *foreign animal proteins*—that is, any animal proteins other than your own. Your immune system is *not* generally watching for plant proteins, because plants (except fungi) are not going to infect you. So animal proteins may act as inflammators, unbalancing and weakening your immune system. An unbalanced or weakened immune system may also be on the lookout for certain plant proteins that can cause an allergic reaction.

Your ideal is a balance of pro- and anti-inflammatory forces, with a powerful yet stable immune system. Studies indicate that animal proteins in food may lead to higher levels of inflammatory markers, while plant foods reduce excessive inflammation.

The Perfect Formula Diet has a role as one key factor in achieving balance. You can reduce both the everyday inflammators from food and strengthen your defensive forces so menaces to your health are overcome more quickly. Don't miss your chance to improve your health through simple, enjoyable lifestyle changes.

CHAPTER 15

Perfect Puzzle Completed

You've come a long way in understanding since you started this book. You now have many puzzle pieces to help you understand, prevent, and overcome chronic disease. While inflammation may have one leading role on center stage, other players—all related to your food choices—can contribute to a downward health spiral.

The Perfect Formula Diet promotes balance and good health in an abundance of ways—that is why it is so potent. Your Perfect Body is complex and no single process can, by itself, explain all illness. So, you'll benefit from appreciating a more complete picture while new studies continue to cast light on these complex processes.

Another Corner Of The Puzzle

Another leading player number contributing to chronic illness is a little-known hormone called insulin-like growth factor-1, or IGF-1 for short. Your liver makes IGF-1, which is a key controller of cell division and death, energy metabolism, body size, lifespan, and overall body functioning.

Proteins you eat significantly raise your level of IGF-1—sometimes to potentially dangerous levels. This is most strongly demonstrated for cow's milk proteins, but all animal proteins have this effect.

Some researchers have noted that it makes sense that cow's milk would raise IGF-1 levels because the function of this milk is to stimulate and maintain fast growth in calves, whose weight increases 10 times in just 8 months. This would be equivalent to a 7-pound newborn baby ballooning to 70 pounds at 8 months old. Humans are just not meant to grow that fast! The IGF-1 in cow's milk is identical to human IGF-1.

While soy proteins can increase IGF-1 to some extent if eaten to excess in concentrated form, other plant proteins either have no effect or actually lower IGF-1. Other variables, including estrogen and other hormones, zinc, growth hormone, and other growth factors, affect the amount of IGF-1 your body produces.

Some studies indicate that eating more calories also raises IGF-1 levels, but other research concludes the risk is not related to total calories consumed.

Scientists have extensively studied IGF-1 in relation to chronic disease and aging. IGF-1 stimulates cells to absorb amino acids and blood sugar and make even more proteins and sugars. Other growth regulators include insulin, growth hormone, IGF-2 and proteins that bind to both IGF-1 and IGF-2.

Stimulating Cancer Cells And Other Unwise Pursuits

Scientists agree that chronic inflammation from certain viruses, bacteria, chronic irritation (for example, from excess stomach acid splashing on the esophagus), and other inflammators can lead to cancer. This prolonged inflammation can damage your cells, including genetic material (DNA), and spark the original development of cancer.

Even without a specific identifiable cause, chronic inflammation encourages the development, proliferation, and spread of many types of cancer, including colon, stomach, esophageal, lung, liver, breast, cervical, ovarian, and pancreatic. Any chronic inflammation is one trigger for cancer and may facilitate its growth.

IGF-1 is key to understanding how chronic inflammation is the soil for malignant growth.

The inflammatory process stimulates IGF-1 production in order to speed repair of damaged tissues. Once in circulation in your body, though, IGF-1 amplifies inflammation as a contributor to chronic illness—especially cancer, the most feared chronic illness.

Numerous studies have demonstrated that higher levels of IGF-1 significantly raise your risk of developing several malignancies, including colon, breast, lung, melanoma, and prostate cancer. Cancer cells respond to lower amounts of growth factors than normal cells need.

IGF-1 nurtures cancer cells by stimulating them to grow faster. Just as deadly, IGF-1 blocks apoptosis, the normal cell death that prunes old or defective cells and prevents damaged cells from reproducing. Without high levels of IGF-1 related to chronic inflammation, many cancer cells would simply self-destruct. IGF-1 also encourages new blood vessels that supply the tumor with the nutrients needed to proliferate and facilitates the spread of tumors.

The drug Tamoxifen, for example, works to reduce the incidence of breast cancer by making the action of IGF-1 on breast tissue weaker. *Wouldn't it make sense to lower IGF-1 levels naturally by eating an animal-free diet?*

The Right Amount Of IGF-1

High levels of IGF-1 may play a role in other illnesses as well, although this isn't as well studied. IGF-1 stimulates lung tissue remodeling that precedes asthma. It also encourages the growth of tiny blood vessels to nourish plaque, clogging your 70,000-mile arterial traffic jam even more.

A European researcher, Dr. Melnik, urges scientists to investigate the possibility that cow's milk proteins can permanently shift IGF-1 levels upward. Such unnaturally high levels of this hormone throughout life could facilitate the development of chronic illness including cardiovascular disease, acne, diabetes, obesity, and neurodegenerative diseases.

Here's what your Perfect Body was designed for. The natural, healthy trajectory of IGF-1 levels is to increase slowly from birth to puberty, spike in the teen years, and decline in adulthood. If this process is reshaped from its biological ideal, high levels of IGF-1 can accelerate the aging process itself. Some researchers have looked at reducing IGF-1 levels as a strategy to increase longevity. People who survive in generally good health to age 100 or more tend to have lower IGF-1 levels than other older people.

You may be wondering by now what positive function IGF-1 plays for you. After all, your Perfect Body would not manufacture a hormone with no beneficial role. A proper level of IGF-1 is critical to survival, supporting growth in your younger years and maintenance of muscle strength in your older years.

The catch is this—IGF-1 works best in this useful way when you are in a balanced inflammatory state. This is a classic example that no one aspect of your body can be understood apart from the whole complex system. Think about that for a minute.

If chronic inflammation is high, then IGF-1 doesn't have the biological activity it's supposed to. Unfortunately, while IGF-1 loses much of its worthwhile activity when inflammation is elevated, it still stimulates the growth of cancer.

Chronic inflammation raises the risk of loss of skeletal muscle cells and general body wasting (cachexia is the scientific name for this) regardless of diet because muscle protein metabolism degrades. Cachexia is an unwelcome accompaniment of many chronic inflammatory illnesses, such as chronic obstructive pulmonary disease (COPD), cancer, liver cirrhosis, chronic heart failure, and end-stage kidney disease.

For example, burn victims—who are in a state of massive inflammation—suffer skeletal muscle breakdown even if they're fed high levels of protein. Their IGF-1 has become largely nonfunctional in its ability to maintain muscle. As another illustration, kidney disease patients who are supplemented with amino acids during dialysis still had a net loss of amino acids from their muscles as a result of chronic inflammation.

Being in a balanced inflammatory state supports the formation of lean, attractive, strong muscle. By choosing the Perfect Formula

Diet, you maximize your ability to attain enviable outcome while avoiding the dangers of illegal drugs and hormones to artificially achieve a similar end.

Turn It Around!

You'll probably not be surprised to learn that the Perfect Formula Diet is one powerful factor for getting your IGF-1 functionality back on track.

- Your diet will be free of the animal proteins that most strongly elevate IGF-1.
- You will be eating the Perfect Foods that normalize IGF-1 levels, promote the self-destruction of malignant and other defective or damaged cells, and support the preservation of muscle tissue in older people.
- Since chronic inflammation is likely to be reduced, you won't need so much IGF-1 to maintain muscle mass and healthy functioning. Your body will be able to do more with less. The only losers are any malignant cells, now deprived of their greatest supporter.

To keep IGF-1 at an optimal level, eat only *whole* soy foods such as edamame (green soybeans), roasted soy nuts, tofu, tempeh, soy-milk, soy yogurt, and products made with such whole or minimally processed ingredients. These foods are not concentrated sources of soy protein. A couple of servings a day are enough (you can also eat other beans instead of soy if you prefer, or just eat potatoes instead).

Avoid *isolated soy protein powder* (and foods made with this ingredient) as concentrated soy protein can raise IGF-1 levels. This *soy protein powder* is a manufactured food that strips only the protein out of the whole bean, creating a substance for which your Perfect Body is not designed.

Another promising area for scientists to explore is the relation-ship between IGF-1 and weight gain. You know how hungry teens are; this is the age group with the naturally highest IGF-1 levels.

Might IGF-1 stimulate the appetite so you have the food to fuel growth? If you're above your Perfect Weight, this is still another reason to reduce elevated IGF-1 levels. If you're an adult, you don't want to fool your body into thinking you need to eat as much as a teenager.

Insulin: A Fresh Path To Understanding

Insulin and IGF-1 are related hormones, as you probably guessed from IGF-1's full name (insulin-like growth factor-1). Insulin also acts as a growth factor encouraging cells, including malignant cells, to divide.

You have undoubtedly heard a distorted, incomplete story about insulin many times from the popular media, which often wrongly blames "carbs" for high insulin levels and insulin resistance.

While eating Perfect Foods leads to lower levels of fasting insulin (the level of insulin several hours after you last ate), people who eat more animal proteins have significantly higher levels of fasting insulin. Your body secretes more insulin when you have higher levels of amino acids, broken down from proteins in your diet, as well as when you eat more sugar. After eating animal protein, your insulin levels may remain elevated for hours.

Eating too much protein can make your body hyper-responsive to glucose, so when you do eat any sugar, you release more insulin than people who eat less protein. At the same time, the ability of your cells to absorb glucose falls. The concentration of insulin in your blood rises both after a single meal high in protein and when you eat too much protein over the long term.

When you keep insulin levels low with a whole plant foods diet, your body burns both glucose and fat for fuel. This condition is conducive to weight loss.

More Supporting Players

Now you understand the crucial roles of inflammation, IGF-1, and insulin in determining health. Other players also have a key part in health outcomes, either directly or through their effect on inflammatory balance. These factors include:

- Oxidation and free radicals
- Certain fats: omega-3 and omega-6 fatty acids, trans fats, and arachidonic acid
- Hormones, especially estrogen in cows' milk and in other animal foods
- Advanced glycation end products (AGEs) and heterocyclic amines (HCAs)

Read on to better understand how each of these actors is related to your health and food choices. This impressive list of health-related factors explains much chronic illness, but is not intended to be a complete description of the cause of every illness you may develop. Scientists make new discoveries every day, so stay alert and be prepared for evolving information.

Rusting From The Inside

Oxygen is an element that's quick to react with other substances to release energy. Oxygen makes things burn. Oxygen makes things rust.

Chemical reactions between oxygen and our foods generate energy that fuels life. Because these metabolic processes release so much energy, they can be difficult to control. Our bodies have intricate mechanisms to assure that when food combines with oxygen, harm from this normal metabolism is minimized. Unfortunately, there's no way to bring the adverse consequences to zero.

Some of the oxygen molecules that combine with food in your body are left with unpaired electrons. These electrically charged oxygen molecules, called reactive oxygen species or free radicals, cause havoc with normal cells. This damage leads to inflammation and can hasten the aging process, cardiovascular disease, malignancy, severe muscle weakness, and other chronic illnesses. Oxidative damage to your joints can be a significant cause of arthritis.

In addition to normal metabolism, environmental pollutants, radiation, some chemicals and drugs, certain metals in foods (such as iron), and inflammation itself can generate free radicals. Thus your body needs effective and constant defense against these destructive molecules.

Your Food Choices Can Fight Free Radicals

The vitamins and phytochemicals in Perfect Foods are powerful antioxidants, neutralizing free radicals quickly before they have a chance to cause significant injury. Herbs and spices are particularly effective sources of concentrated antioxidants, which is a key reason the Perfect Formula Diet is based on foods flavored with these delicious ingredients.

Reactive oxygen species can sever your DNA, the repository of your genetic code and master control for all the proteins you synthesize. A European study of 161 women found that, in those who ate meat, oxidative damage to DNA increased markedly between ages 30 and 60. However, older women who choose a meat-free diet had DNA as intact as women 30 to 40 years younger, likely protecting them from health-related effects of aging.

In addition to causing disease and damaging your DNA, free radicals also promote skin aging and wrinkles. A multinational study found that Perfect Foods protect the skin, while meat, dairy, butter, margarine, and sugar were associated with increased skin damage.

The robust antioxidant protection from Perfect Foods is another reason that the Perfect Formula Diet can be your path to Perfect Health (not to mention smoother skin). While Perfect Foods have this protective force, many studies of *isolated* vitamins and phytochemicals have found little to no antioxidant protection from such supplemental pills and liquids.

Fatty Factors In Inflammation

Both omega-3 and omega-6 fatty acids are essential to life. Plants alone make these building blocks (*not* fish, who get their omega-3s from the wild plants they eat). Establishing the optimal *ratio* of omega-3 to omega-6 fatty acids in your diet is a cornerstone of keeping your body in balance. In fact, while your body does require omega-3 and omega-6 fatty acids, the amount required is small—less than 2% of the calories you eat.

While omega-3s are generally anti-inflammatory in their biological activity, omega-6s are generally pro-inflammatory. There are fairly equal amounts of omega-3s and omega-6s in your brain, and eating approximately the same amounts of these fats is important to avoid mental health problems, including depression and memory problems.

Concentrated omega-6 fatty acids in vegetable oils—in bottled oils, margarine, and foods cooked or coated with these oils—add to your inflammatory burden. The fatty acid ratio for citizens of developed countries changed for the worse after 1913, when readily available refined vegetable oils were introduced.

Wild plants—the original foods that humans are designed for—are naturally higher in omega-3s than plants cultivated on farms. Since you likely eat few wild plants, you need an extra boost of omega-3s from Perfect Foods to keep your omega-3 to omega-6 ratio at its ideal level. Omega-6 fatty acids are abundant in many foods, and you don't have to worry about getting enough of them on the Perfect Formula Diet.

The easiest, most inexpensive way to accomplish your omega-3 boost is to eat two tablespoons a day of ground flax seeds, which are an excellent source of omega-3s, as well as fiber and cancer-fighting phytochemicals. You can sprinkle the ground flax seeds on whole grain cereal, oatmeal, salad, soups, smoothies, or any other food you like. The taste is quite mild and pleasant, and your monthly cost should be only a few dollars.

You need to grind the flax seed before your body can use it because of its hard hull. The best way to do this is in a coffee grinder. You can buy flax seeds already ground, but be careful you don't buy flax meal, which has the beneficial omega-3s already removed.

You might have heard a lot of hype about fish oil as a source of omega-3s. One of the many problems with this is that fish have only as many omega-3s as the wild foods they ate. Farmed fish generally do not get to eat wild plants.

Omega-3s in general oxidize and become rancid rapidly. Fish oil can quickly break down and deteriorate in your body, causing harmful oxidation. A summary of 89 studies on fish oil found that it doesn't increase life span.

A group of Canadian scientists forcefully demonstrate that there are not nearly enough fish in the planet's severely depleted waters to supply all people with omega-3s, and the thoughtless quest to ignore this basic fact is driving ever more destructive and unsustainable fishing practices. The fat, mercury, and pollutants in fish oil are far from health foods, and more than 90% of large fish in the ocean are gone because of over-fishing and pollution.

The omega-3s in ground flax seed stay fresh longer than fish oil because of the many protective antioxidants in this Perfect Food. As an alternative, you can try capsules of omega-3s from marine algae, which is naturally high in this fat. Cost is one disadvantage of this solution, but you may find it more convenient.

Researchers are a long way from determining whether too much omega-3, just as too much omega-6, can be harmful. Excess omega-3s may get turned into saturated fat or spur inflammatory factors. For that reason, you may prefer to be safe and get your omega-3s from food instead of supplements. However, if you are still consuming bottled vegetable oils or margarine in significant quantities, it may be a good idea to take the algae-based omega-3 supplements to balance the omega-6s in the oil. Further research is needed to address this question.

Another inflammatory fat, which is just about eliminated in the Perfect Formula Diet, is trans fat. All dairy fats and meats naturally contain some trans fats, as do many manufactured foods. These substances, which should be vigorously avoided, are usually called hydrogenated or partially hydrogenated vegetable oils on food labels. You need to read ingredients instead of just looking at a label and relaxing if it says zero trans fats. This is because small amounts of these dangerous substances can be rounded down to zero on food labels.

According the National Academy of Sciences, the tolerable upper intake level for trans fats from a health standpoint is zero. While trans fats are best known for contributing to cardiovascular disease, these substances interfere with the functioning of cells throughout your body, especially in your brain.

Arachidonic acid (AA) is an additional inflammatory fatty acid that occurs mostly in animal foods such as meat, dairy products, and eggs. Your body can also convert the omega-6 fats in vegetable oils to AA.

Substances released when AA is metabolized contribute to the growth of cancer, blood clots, narrowing of blood vessels, allergies, and arthritis. While some AA is necessary for normal functioning, your body can make its own AA and dietary excess is inflammatory. Following the Perfect Formula Diet will drastically reduce the amount of AA that you eat—still another way of supporting your Perfect Health.

Cows Must Give Birth To Secrete Milk

Dairy cows, like all mammals, produce milk only after they have given birth to a baby. To get the maximum milk, dairy owners keep cows pregnant as much as possible. They take the calves away from their mothers within hours of birth, creating unimaginable distress for both the cow and her baby. The mother cow is then impregnated again as soon as possible, and the milk meant for the calf is sucked into machines to be processed and sold.

This impacts your health. The biologically active reproductive hormones you ingest with dairy and other animal foods may increase your cancer risk. Estrogen promotes hormone-related cancers, such as prostate and testicular cancer in men and breast, endometrial, and ovarian cancers in women.

Dairy cows, like all pregnant mammals, produce high levels of estrogen to maintain their pregnancies. In fact, glands in the cow's udder secrete estrogen. This hormone is essential for the animal's preparation to nurse her baby. The cows with the highest levels of estrogen in the blood supply to their udders produce the most milk.

This estrogen filters into cows' milk, and you consume this hormone, which is very similar to human estrogen, when you eat or drink dairy products. Seventy-five percent of commercial milk—the kind you buy in grocery stores—comes from pregnant cows. Skim milk is even higher in estrogen than whole milk.

You easily absorb the estrogen in dairy products during digestion. Studies show that drinking cows' milk raises circulating estrogen levels in both men and women. Pregnant cows also produce more progesterone, another reproductive hormone, which can also be absorbed by people.

Sixty to eighty percent of all estrogens that people eat come, on average, from milk and dairy products. Eggs are also another significant source of dietary estrogen.

Even so-called "beef" cows—raised for their muscles instead of their milk—often are implanted with natural and synthetic hormones to make them grow faster. These hormones can also lead to undesirable health consequences for people who eat the resulting meat. Pigs, chickens, and fish also contain steroid hormones.

The powerful animal foods industry may try to fool you with hype about supposed harmful effects from phytoestrogens (plant versions of estrogen) in soy and other plant foods. The fact is that soy has feeble estrogenic effects that can help women make up for too little estrogen or partially block the impact of too much estrogen.

Remember, soy is a plant, and plants have very different reproductive pathways than mammals do. You would do much better to avoid the potent estrogens in animal foods—by following the Perfect Formula Diet!

AGEs and HCAs: What Can Happen When You Cook
Advanced glycation end products (AGEs) are inflammatory toxic molecules in food, and are especially harmful for people with diabetes. Cooking animal and plant foods at high temperatures (for example by grilling or frying) produces AGEs, especially if refined sugars are added.

AGEs accumulate in your body, promoting chronic disease and making it harder for your tissues to do their job. For example, the AGEs that collect in cartilage make it more likely that you will develop osteoarthritis in the affected joint.

AGEs also contribute to the development of Alzheimer's disease, high blood pressure, cardiovascular disease, cataracts, kidney failure, and erectile dysfunction. For type 2 diabetes patients, those with the highest levels of AGEs (measured with a skin test) are more likely to develop diabetic complications, such as cardiovascular disease and neuropathy.

By now you won't be surprised to learn that AGEs are found in greatest abundance in animal foods, especially if cooked at high temperatures. The foods highest in AGEs include broiled hot dogs and broiled or oven fried chicken and fish. Cheese and egg yolks are also high in AGEs.

Perfect Foods have the least amount of AGEs per forkful. However, French fries, broiled tofu, and roasted nuts can form a significant amount of AGEs as well. The lesson is that, to minimize AGEs, eat lots of Perfect Foods that are raw, boiled, steamed, or otherwise cooked at a relatively low temperature.

You've probably also heard of heterocyclic amines (HCAs), a class of cancer-causing substances that forms when meat (including fish) is cooked at high temperatures. HCAs can bind directly to your

DNA, causing it to mutate and eventually produce malignant cells. HCAs, which form most prolifically when animal foods (especially chicken) are broiled, fried, or grilled, have been specifically linked to higher risk for colorectal cancer. This is still one more reason that an animal-free diet is the basis for Perfect Health.

Your Bones Are More Than Calcium

Given the intense media focus on osteoporosis, learning more about your 206 bones is essential for intelligent response to this hype. Your bones are living tissue with nerves and blood vessels. Connective tissue, reinforced by protein fibers, forms the groundwork of your bones, which have an intricate anatomy. This includes an external hard component with a cylindrical structure and a softer core with a honeycomb structure.

Minerals that your bones store include not just calcium, but also sodium, magnesium, phosphate, and others. Maintaining the optimum level of these minerals is vital for the proper functioning of every cell in your body; your bones serve as inventory central. Minerals are stored mostly in the spaces of the honeycomb structure of your bones.

Cells called osteoblasts, which form bone tissue, and osteoclasts, which break down old, weak, or diseased bone, constantly remodel your skeleton. This complex process depends on a host of vitamins, inflammatory substances, and hormones to keep the right balance of bone formation and break down.

This remodeling is not just healthy—it's essential! Your bones need to be able to constantly regenerate, clear out dead or malfunctioning cells, heal if broken, and change their shape and strength to respond to environmental demands. For example, putting weight on bones encourages new tissue to form, while inactivity leads your body to get rid of unneeded bone mass.

Bone dissolution and bone formation cannot be separated because they're two sides of the same coin. As old bone breaks down into its component amino acids, minerals, and enzymes, the substances released are the building blocks for constructing strong new bone.

Thicker Bones Are Not Necessarily Stronger Bones

You care how easily your bones fracture; how thick they are is immaterial. You want bones that are strong and durable, resisting breakage when subject to inevitable forces of gravity and mechanical stress. So what role do calcium and heavily mineralized bones play in achieving this goal?

Infants are born with little calcium in their skeletons. Instead, young children's bones, made of flexible cartilage, tend to bend rather than fracture when subjected to force. This is the first hint that calcium is not the most vital factor in durable bones.

In fact, the skeletal problem caused by pure lack of minerals is called rickets in children and osteomalacia in adults. These conditions are usually caused by vitamin D deficiency or problems with vitamin D metabolism, *not* by a calcium shortage.

Other bone problems show that mineral-thick bone is not necessarily stronger. Paget's disease is a relatively common inflammatory condition in older people in Western countries. Bone mass increases, but the thick bone is structurally weak and unsound. Osteopetrosis is a rare hereditary condition in which the cells that break down bone don't work properly. Again, the resulting bone is hard and stone-like, but extremely brittle and easily fractured.

Fluoride stimulates bone formation, but the incidence of fractures may rise because the resulting bone is weak. Diabetics tend to have higher bone mineral density, but still have a significantly increased risk of hip fracture. Supplements of calcium and vitamin D can raise bone mineral density without reducing the risk of hip, spine, or total fractures. A study of about 200 people with an average age of 75 found no significant association between a person's bone mineral density and whether he or she had suffered a vertebral fracture.

A study of 73 women and 82 men found that people could not actively absorb more than 500 mg a day of calcium, and this was plenty for people who ate little salt and protein. Those fed more protein and salt used about 700 mg of calcium per day. Beyond that amount, the participants simply excreted extra calcium. Another study found that, for people with adequate vitamin D, no more than 800 mg of calcium a day was necessary to maintain their bodies' calcium stores.

Researchers compared a group of 105 Buddhist nuns on an animal-free diet with 105 women of similar ages in their communities. Although the nuns consumed an average of 330 mg of calcium per day, and had been on a plant-based diet for an average of 33 years, these women suffered no ill effects on their bone health.

If you're still concerned about calcium, be aware that acidic animal proteins cause your body to leach calcium from your bones to neutralize the dangerous acid. Plants, which need calcium for essential metabolic processes, are rich in this mineral, so you don't need animal foods to get enough. You can get your calcium where the cows get theirs—from plants.

Inflammation Can Dissolve Your Bones

If you want to understand the damage inflammation can inflict on your bones, just look in the mirror and open your mouth. In severe gum disease, called periodontitis, inflammation from bacterial infection in your mouth dissolves the bone anchoring your teeth. Scientists need to thoroughly illuminate the mechanism for this so we can see how it applies to chronic inflammation and brittle bones throughout your body.

The truth is that calcium and other minerals cannot even get into your bone without a matrix of living tissue to support their storage. Strong, fracture-resistant bone results from the natural process of selective pruning of old, weak, or damaged bone tissue and the formation of a strong new matrix.

The amount of calcium you consume has virtually nothing to do with this process. Not surprisingly, inflammation does. An excess of both pro- and anti-inflammatory substances contributes to the disruption of vital bone remodeling. Inflammatory substances stimulate osteoclasts to break down your bones—hence the damage to your bone in periodontitis.

Staying in inflammatory balance is the foundation for healthy bones. If you are diagnosed with "osteoporosis," ask your doctor why excessive calcium or drugs that interfere with normal bone metabolism would be beneficial and help you stay in balance. Then you can make more informed decisions about what you want to do to truly decrease your risk of fractures.

The Story Condensed

If you've read Chapters 12 through 15, congratulations! You now have a comprehensive picture of several key determinants of chronic illness and their likely relation to diet. More than most people, you know why you may get sick and how to stay well.

Your body interprets inflammation as an emergency. Normal processes are slowed or shut down and resources are channeled into healing. Muscle doesn't strengthen as it should and bone doesn't grow properly.

While inflammation is perhaps the most critical factor, another leading player in chronic illness is insulin-like growth factor-1 (IGF-1), which encourages cell division and cancer. Both inflammation and animal proteins in food increase your level of IGF-1, while plant proteins generally don't have this effect.

Recall that, with chronic inflammation, your immune system is not functioning at its peak and has a tougher time killing malignant cells. So chronic inflammation may:

- Damage your DNA
- Weaken your immune system
- Encourage malignant cells to thrive with IGF-1 and a nourishing blood supply
- Undermine the process of normal death of abnormal cells

These processes add up to a quadruple blow to your chances for survival from cancer.

Proteins, as well as carbohydrates, stimulate your body to release insulin.

While oxidation can harm you and cause wrinkles, Perfect Foods contain powerful antioxidants that cannot be duplicated by supplements.

The best place to get your anti-inflammatory omega-3 fatty acids is ground flax seeds, not fish oil.

Dairy cows, kept almost constantly pregnant, produce high levels of cancer-promoting estrogen that gets into their milk, and into you when you consume dairy products.

Advanced glycation end products (AGEs) form in foods, especially animal products, cooked at high temperatures. AGEs are inflammatory and contribute to chronic illness.

Your bones are living tissue that is constantly being remodeled. Strong bone results from the natural process of selective pruning of old, weak, or damaged bone and the formation of strong new tissue. An excess of both pro- and anti-inflammatory substances contributes to the disruption of vital bone remodeling. Staying in inflammatory balance is the foundation for strong, durable, fracture-resistant bones.

The Perfect Formula Diet promotes Perfect Health in so many ways, drastically reducing the risk of chronic illness. At the same time, Perfect Foods are the foundation of balance—the best way to keep all parts of your Perfect Body strong and thriving.

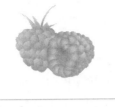

CHAPTER 16

Perfect Planet

Just as your body is naturally perfect, so too our planet is naturally perfect. And just as you harm your body by working against it instead of with it, we degrade our planet by disrupting the complex web of life, wiping out species, and drenching the land, sea, and air with toxic chemicals.

The dangerous substances polluting our planet are inflammators once they get into your body. Just like any other inflammator, these pollutants can lead to chronic illness and death. Chemicals that act as hormone disruptors can also make you gain weight.

Your health and the well-being of your children, grandchildren, nieces, nephews, and all current and future generations are inextricably bound up with the health of the earth. Humans cannot thrive for long on a deteriorating planet, although short-term techno-fixes can temporarily hide these interrelationships.

The good news is that you have the power to heal both your body and the planet. Your most powerful tool in both endeavors is the same: the Perfect Formula Diet. Animal foods are likely the chief source of dangerous chemical pollutants in your body and your family's bodies. Raising animals for food fouls air and water, aggravates resource scarcity and high prices, and is the origin of staggering amounts of environmental pollutants.

Chemical Waste Disposal—In Your Body!

More than 85,000 industrial chemicals are used in the U.S., with more than 2,000 new chemicals added to this roster annually. Scientists don't know how most of these chemicals affect humans (animal studies add no useful insight into this question).

As these chemicals leach, dissolve, burn, or otherwise get into the environment, many wind up inside of you. The Centers for Disease Control reports that Americans have an average of 116 manmade chemicals or pollutants in their bodies. And these are just the chemicals that scientists have searched for and detected—there may be many more.

Close Your Eyes, But It Won't Just Go Away

Persistent organic pollutants (POPs) are deadly. People manufacture these chemicals for uses including pesticides, herbicides, building materials, and other industrial and agricultural applications. Some industrial processes and combustion generate other dangerous POPs. Among the most well-known are PCBs, DDT, dioxins, and PBDEs (flame retardants).

The following dangerous properties make POPs especially hazardous to humans and wildlife.

- High toxicity, with adverse effects including death, disease, and birth defects. Cancer, nervous system damage, behavior problems, Parkinson's disease, reproductive disorders, immune system disruption and autoimmune disorders, diabetes, and allergies can all result from exposure to POPs.
- Ability to disrupt normal endocrine processes, which can cause reproductive and immune problems over multiple generations as well as weight gain. These endocrine disrupters, which affect estrogen, thyroid, and other hormonal functions, are the enemy of Perfect Weight.
- Highly stable in the environment, resisting breakdown and maintaining their toxic effects for decades or longer.

- Highly stable in the body, resisting breakdown and excretion by normal protective processes and causing progressive harm over time.
- Transferred from mother to nursing infant via breast milk.
- Easily transported through the atmosphere, ocean, and rivers far from their place of origin.
- Dissolve and are stored in fat, so accumulate in the tissues of animals and become more concentrated higher on the food chain (when animals eat other animals contaminated with POPs). This process of "bioaccumulation" can magnify POP concentration up to 70,000 times more than the original amount in the environment. Creatures most at risk from this process are fish, predatory birds and mammals, and humans.
- Widely used, with feeble regulation and enforcement considering the serious hazards to health and ecological integrity.

Watch Out!

POPs are far from the only environmental threats to your health. Lead and mercury, among other heavy metals, are dangerous and also accumulate in your body, posing a special hazard to the young. Think about that for a minute.

Numerous prescription drugs, including antibiotics, anticonvulsants, mood-altering chemicals, and sex hormones contaminate the drinking water of at least 41 million Americans. These drugs are dumped directly into water or are excreted by patients without being metabolized. And this is only the beginning of the catalogue of dangerous pollutants.

Tanning skin from animals to make leather generates additional significant pollutants, including salt, hydrogen sulfide, chromium, lime, and particles of dead animals, into local waterways. Without such a heavy infusion of chemicals, skin begins to decay soon after death, along with the rest of an animal's body.

Environmental pollutants can actually change the way in which your genes are expressed! For example, pesticides, air pollutants, industrial chemicals, and heavy metals can all distort how your genes make your body function. These chemically-caused changes in how genes work can increase your risk of developing cancer, diabetes, obesity, infertility, respiratory disease, allergies, Parkinson's disease, and Alzheimer's disease.

Environmental cardiology, an emerging medical field, builds on evidence that exposure to a variety of pollutants has a substantial impact on heart disease. Effects of these hazardous substances include atherosclerosis, constricted blood vessels, variable heart rate, and high blood pressure leading potentially to heart disease, congestive heart failure, heart attack, arrhythmias, and stroke.

Chowing Down Chemicals

While dangerous pollutants can make their way into your body through breathing, personal care and household products, and contaminated water, the major source of these potentially deadly substances for most people is animal foods—meat, poultry, fish, and dairy products.

Such animal foods are most likely the source of 89% to 99% of POPs in your body. This is because these chemicals, which are at comparatively low levels in plant foods, bioaccumulate in the fat and milk of animals who eat plants and concentrate in each step up the food chain. Factory farming magnifies this danger by feeding animal remains and fish meal (both of which already have higher levels of POPs than plants) to naturally vegetarian farmed animals to speed weight gain and increase milk production.

A study of U.S. supermarkets found the product most contaminated with PDBE, a class of POPs used as flame retardants, was fish. Meat and dairy products placed second and third in contamination levels. A British study found significantly more PBDEs in animal foods than in plant foods, and concluded that 93% of PDBE exposure was through diet.

Two studies found those on a plant-based diet had lower PDBE levels than most people and, the longer the person was on an animal-free diet, the less PDBEs and dioxin were in their blood. A

Boston study found that the more dairy products and meat a new mother ate, the more PDBEs were likely to be in her breast milk.

While animal foods are likely the chief culprits in flooding your body with chemicals, Perfect Foods encourage detoxification of these environmental contaminants. The fiber in Perfect Foods also helps speed toxic chemicals through and out of your digestive tract.

Organic plant foods have the lowest levels of POPs and will be the most beneficial in clearing your body of a lifetime of toxic accumulations. Children who eat only organic foods have six to nine times less exposure to toxic pesticides than kids on a standard diet. It's best if you thoroughly wash all plant foods to remove surface POPs.

Fishing For Hazards

Food chains are longer in the ocean, lakes, and rivers than on land. The many steps of big fish eating smaller fish and then being eaten themselves results in greater accumulation of POPs in marine creatures.

The toxic heavy metals washed and rained into natural waters also concentrate in the unfortunate creatures exposed to these deadly pollutants. Fish and shellfish are the main source of mercury for humans. In addition to harming the developing brains of unborn and young children, mercury increases the risk of heart attack in adults.

Fish exist at the intersection of water pollution and toxic chemicals in animal foods. Human activity has measurably damaged 96% of the world's oceans through climate destabilization, fishing, pollution, shipping, habitat destruction, and other activities.

The fish remaining in the wild are getting sick from water contaminants. As one example, more than half the brown bullhead catfish studied in the South River in Maryland had skin tumors and another fifth had liver cancer. In the Great Lakes, more than half the population of this species had skin cancer. Multiple studies have found male fish growing eggs because of the effects of endocrine disruptors from pollutants.

Are these animals you want to eat? How healthy are other fish species that may not have been studied so intensively?

Fishing For Extinction

The number of fish gracing our planet is plummeting. Fourteen scientists from around the world studied four years of global data and project that by 2048, people will no longer have any fish left to eat. These scientists observed that the populations of about a third of all fish species have already collapsed. Only about 10% of the large fish in the ocean when modern fishing techniques started are left today.

As any one species declines, other species that are interlinked in the same ecosystem also fade away, making it ever more difficult for the web of life to recover. Bottom trawling, a viciously destructive practice subsidized by short-sighted governments, destroys entire ecosystems by dragging heavy nets and crushing rollers across the sea floor. "Non-target" fish, invertebrates, seabirds, turtles, and marine mammals are destroyed by the ton as people fish. Whales and other creatures get tangled in commercial fishing nets and lobster gear.

If you think these are reasons to eat farmed fish or land animals instead of wild-caught fish, consider these facts. *Three to five pounds of wild fish are needed for feed to produce one pound of farmed fish.*

Up to 95% of wild young salmon migrating past fish farms die after infestation by sea lice that thrive in the crowded fish farms. Fish are often "farmed" in estuaries and other habitats that are prime breeding grounds for wild fish—until destroyed by fish farms.

Factory farmed land animals, including pigs and chickens, are fed up to half of wild-caught fish. This practice further devastates wild fish populations and results in more dangerous contamination of meat with the heavy metals and POPs from fish.

If you eat any animal foods at all, there is no way around it. You are directly contributing to emptying the oceans and devastating our planet's ability to support life. At the same time, you are likely flooding your body with chemical inflammators.

Children And Men At Risk

Babies around the world are born with hazardous chemicals in their bodies. Tests of the umbilical cord blood of 10 randomly selected babies born in the U.S. in 2004 found these infants had been subjected to an average 200 industrial chemicals and pollutants before birth. Pesticides, consumer product ingredients, flame retardants, and waste products from burning coal, gasoline, and garbage were among the substances detected.

Prenatal exposure to POPs and other environment pollutants may lead to both immediate and long-term functional abnormalities and illnesses. These include neurodevelopmental issues and mental illness, reduced intelligence, lower growth rate, cancer, diabetes, and endocrine, immune system, and hormonal problems. The rate at which kids develop cancer increased by 27% between 1975 and 2002. Exposure to toxic industrial chemicals before birth and in early infancy may be sparking neurodevelopmental disorders at epidemic levels because the developing brain is so vulnerable to even low levels of pollutants.

Autism, specifically, may be related to prenatal brain damage from environmental toxins such as mercury and other heavy metals, certain medications, smoking, and chlorinated solvents. Mercury, which gets into people of all ages mostly through fish, may disrupt hormones and cause premature birth as well as directly poison the baby's developing nervous system.

During the last several decades, baby boys have suffered more than twice the incidence of developmental reproductive abnormalities. During this same period, sperm counts in normal adult men have fallen by half. Between 1975 and 2002, the rate of testicular cancer increased by 66%.

Scientists believe these male reproductive problems are likely related to high exposure of the fetus to estrogen, which can flood pregnant women's bodies from cow's milk, prescription hormones excreted into the water supply, and the estrogen-like activity of POPs.

Breathing: Not Optional

You determine what you eat, but will have a more difficult time controlling the air you breathe. Unfortunately, the very atmosphere you depend on for survival is filled with hazardous wastes that are inflammators once they enter your body. Globally, air pollution is the 13th leading cause of death. Air pollution can activate or intensify the expression of inflammatory genes leading to respiratory disease.

Fine particulates from diesel exhaust and other fossil fuel combustion are especially dangerous, carried all over your body in your blood. The Environmental Protection Agency estimates that particulate air pollution kills 60,000 people each year in the U.S. alone. In developed areas of Europe, air pollution from traffic kills more people than auto accidents.

These tiny particles and other pollutants in the air are inflammators sparking systemic inflammation, and are especially dangerous for cardiovascular and respiratory health. Such air-borne waste is also a risk factor for preterm birth, low birth weight, death of the fetus, reduced learning ability, hormone disruption, ear infections, and brain inflammation.

While you can't buy clean air in the supermarket, don't give up on your quest to eliminate air pollution as a source of chronic illness. In the short term, you can take common-sense measures such as driving less, living and working away from major roads to the extent possible, giving a wide berth to anyone who is smoking, and not exercising in polluted areas.

For the long term, you can join and become active in environmental groups working to clean up the air, writing and calling politicians and regulators, and making your family and friends aware of the issue.

By sticking to the Perfect Formula Diet, you will optimize your health and your body's ability to cope with air pollution you can't avoid. You will also clean the air. This happens when you reduce ammonia, hydrogen sulfide, and fine dust from manure waste on factory farms by sticking to whole plant foods.

The Story Condensed

The health of humans and the health of our planet cannot be separated. You can't be any healthier than the environment you live in. You can't make these problems go away by ignoring them.

To stay lean and healthy, avoid manmade chemicals, heavy metals, and air-borne pollutants that are increasingly flooding your environment. These deadly inflammators can cause disabling chronic illness and disrupt your body's natural hormonal processes, leading to weight gain and potential reproductive problems.

The surest way to protect your naturally Perfect Body is to follow the Perfect Formula Diet. This eating plan both eliminates the animal foods that are the chief source of many dangerous pollutants and ups your intake of Perfect Foods to speed detoxification.

Just as important, by reducing the demand for animal foods, you safeguard future generations and the planet itself. You play a significant role in battling pollution:

- Eliminating factory farm run-off
- Stopping air pollution from manure waste and transport of farmed animals
- Halting the use of pesticides, herbicides, and fertilizer used to grow animal feed
- Preventing further devastation of fish populations and destruction of marine habitat

The next chapter, *Perfect Home*, gives additional suggestions for making sure the only substances in your body are the ones that were designed to be there.

CHAPTER 17

Perfect Home

You can't shampoo your way out of arthritis or heart disease no matter how chemical-free your product is. Diet is a more fundamental factor in determining chronic illness and the major driver for improving your health and reducing your weight.

However, if you're still encountering health challenges after sticking to the Perfect Formula Diet, hidden threats in your home and everyday products could be significant contributing factors. While you probably recognize the danger from large-scale environmental disasters, you may not be aware that you're chronically exposed to low levels of toxic chemicals that may have a *cumulative* effect.

Your skin is like a sponge, absorbing the creams, lotions, perfumes, shampoos, soaps, cleaning products, and so on that you rub into or put onto it. In addition, the vapors from products that you can smell, whether labeled "fragrance" or not, are absorbed into your blood through your lungs. So you're putting many more chemicals into your body than might seem evident at first glance. You're probably not surprised to learn that government agencies' oversight of these products is minimal and absurdly inadequate.

Most Americans experience more air pollution indoors than they do outdoors. Slashing the toxic chemicals in your living environment and personal care products means your naturally Perfect

Body is subject to fewer inflammators and reduced hormone disruption. Manifestations of inflammation from exposure to indoor chemicals include weight gain, respiratory issues, fatigue, headaches, difficulty concentrating or remembering, rashes, itching, muscle and joint aches, menstrual difficulties, and cancer.

Cleaning up your living environment and personal care choices is a relatively simple step, since you're often just substituting natural choices for those with long lists of chemical ingredients. This switch usually involves minimal lifestyle disruption or inconvenience. You may need to shop in different stores for some products, or you can find them online.

Join the surging ranks of shoppers whose top priorities include using nontoxic products. Even in the 2008 economic downturn, 70% of consumers were willing to pay more for healthy alternatives. Another survey of more than 7,700 consumers showed that 87% were concerned about how their product choices impacted the environment and society.

What's At Stake?

More than 80,000 chemicals are used by industry; scientists have only minimal understanding of the human health effects of the vast majority of these. In addition, manmade chemicals interact with each other and those interactions have unknown effects.

A European study on identical twins separated early in life found that cancer risk of adopted children is closer to that of their adoptive parents than it is to their biological parents, indicating the critical role of environmental factors in cancer development. Another study found that exposure to home and garden insecticides or fungicides, including a shampoo used to kill lice, doubled the risk of a child developing acute childhood leukemia.

The Environmental Protection Agency asked eight chemical companies to voluntarily phase out, by 2015, use of the chemical perfluorooctanoic acid (PFOA), which is linked to cancer risk. This substance, used to make plastics more resistant to fire, grease, and stains, is used in artificially coated cookware, fabrics, leather, auto parts, and microwave popcorn bags, among other applications.

Independent testing of 35 Americans in seven states found every single person tested had at least seven toxic chemicals (out of 20 tested for) in his or her body. These chemicals are linked to birth defects, asthma, cancer, learning disabilities, and other negative health consequences.

Toxic chemicals seldom have only one effect on your body. The same chemicals that raise cancer risk may also cause genetic damage, hormonal disruption, reproductive problems, nervous system damage, and blood and immune system harm. Some personal care products contain multiple ingredients that may raise your risk of cancer and other health problems.

Scientists have found that the more it rains and snows in an area, the more likely children who live there are to become autistic, suggesting an environmental trigger for autism. The researchers were not sure if the kids were gaining protection against autism from being outside during nice weather or if they were harmed from being inside more when the weather was uninviting. Given the level of indoor pollution, the potential damage to kids from this exposure should be thoroughly investigated.

What To Invite Into Your Home

While you have limited control over pollutants in the outdoor environment, you do have control over which products to bring into your house or apartment. Furniture, floor coverings, window coverings, mattresses, and so on are major, infrequent purchases. Before you invest in such items, take the time to research which materials are the least toxic.

Personal care and cleaning products, on the other hand, are small and relatively inexpensive purchases. You can start making healthier choices on your next trip to the store.

Goods such as sheets, pillows, clothing, shower curtains, pots and pans, cups and plates, and silverware cost more than soap but less than a new sofa. Depending on the item, you could make purchases every few months to every few years. Again, do your research and become aware of the chemicals you are inviting into your house and your naturally Perfect Body.

Your first defense, as in selecting food, is to read labels. If the item contains a mystery ingredient you don't recognize and can't pronounce or contains artificial fragrance, keep on shopping. You may need to go to a different store or to the Internet, but nontoxic alternatives are available to you. For example, you can get soaps made only with plant oils, without added chemicals or waste products from processing diseased factory farmed animals.

Another defense is to live more simply. Do you really need all those personal care and cleaning products? Can you substitute glass, ceramic, iron or stainless steel for plastics in bottles, pots, plates, cups, and food storage containers? Can you seal the entrance that bugs use to get into your house instead of spraying insecticides?

In making a selection, whether for a $2 or $2,000 purchase, be aware that manufacturers don't have to list all ingredients on labels. Some items do not even have a label. So additional research may be required. Decide for yourself—how much is your health worth? Do you want to invest a little time now to potentially save yourself some trips later to a doctor's office or hospital or chemotherapy clinic?

The Environmental Working Group (EWG) and Organic Consumers Association are two independent nonprofit organizations devoted to giving you reliable information on chemical-free alternatives for household items. See Chapter 21, *Perfect Resources,* for contact information. You can get more information on ingredients to avoid by checking these organization's sites or searching the web.

Looking Good Inside And Out

EWG tested 20 teenage girls across the U.S. and found that these young women already had a detectable average of 13 potentially hormone-altering chemicals from cosmetics in their bodies. EWG had tested for 16 chemicals in 4 categories:

- Phthalates: may disrupt hormones leading to potential risks to the reproductive and thyroid systems, as well as to increased risk for asthma and allergies in children; are found in fragrances, nail polish, hair products, and other personal care products as well as many plastics (food wraps, toys, building materials, etc.), paint, and pesticides
- Triclosan: used to kill bacteria, may disrupt thyroid and reproductive hormone function and encourage bacterial resistance to antibiotics; is found in "antibacterial" liquid hand soaps, toothpastes, deodorants, face and body washes, kitchen items, and other personal care and household items. Breaks down into toxic chemicals, including dioxin and other persistent organic pollutants, in the environment.
- Parabens: may disrupt hormones by mimicking estrogen and may be carcinogenic; used as a preservative in many cosmetics and body care products including moisturizers, skin cleansers, shampoos, conditioners, sunscreens, deodorants, toothpaste, medications, and many others
- Musks: may disrupt hormones and the body's natural defenses against toxic chemicals and raise cancer risk; used in fragrance for cosmetics and body care products, air fresheners, detergents, fabric softeners, cleaning products, and other household items

In their online shopper's guide to safe cosmetics, EWG lists several other ingredients to avoid, such as sodium lauryl sulfate, formaldehyde, imidazolidinyl urea, and DMDM hydantoin. The shoppers guide is a valuable, free one-page reference sheet, so get it and use it.

Maybe you care about looking good more than about being healthy. But the two are inseparable. If you're using toxic chemicals to make yourself more attractive, the advertised benefits could be flooded by the drawbacks. Although chemical-laden lotions and facial products claim to keep you looking younger, does this make sense to you? Isn't it more likely that artificial ingredients with unpronounceable names will age, wrinkle, and damage your skin?

Clean And Green

Chemicals in household cleaning products are often pro-inflammatory, potentially irritating the respiratory tract and causing headaches, lethargy, confusion, and even irregular heartbeat. A study of more than 3,000 adults found that the more people used cleaning sprays, the more they upped their risk of developing asthma. When exposed to chemical irritants such as tobacco smoke, perfume, and fragrance, 98% of people with asthma and 67% of people with rhinitis developed respiratory inflammation.

A better choice is to buy nontoxic cleaning products that don't contain bleach, ammonia, perfume, or artificial fragrance. Even with these products, use as little as possible and ventilate your work area. By searching the Internet, you can learn to make effective cleaning products from simple ingredients such as lemon juice, baking soda, and vinegar.

If you don't like a smell in your home, it's best to open windows and use fans or air purifiers to get rid of the odor. Air fresheners, scented candles, perfumes, and artificial fragrances can all cause inflammation. Natural plant oils are a way better choice.

For cleaning your clothes, aim to buy apparel you don't need to dry clean. If you must dry clean your clothes, choose a business that uses nonsolvent fluids or at least air out your dry cleaning before bringing it into the house.

Carefully read the labels on all laundry soaps, fabric softeners, dryer sheets, etc. If you can't pronounce or recognize the ingredients, or if the product is artificially scented, shop to find a natural alternative or just dispense with the "extras" (everything other than the soap). Try active enzymes as a non-chemical and extremely effective remedy for laundry stains.

If pest control is your worry, research nontoxic ways to control pests. More and more pest control services offer nontoxic remedies.

More Indoor Spaces

Think about the other indoor environments you spend time in, such as your workplace, stores, hotel rooms, repair shops, and hair or nail salons. Can you detect chemical smells, such as from cleaning or personal care products, paints, or carpets?

Your first line of defense is avoidance. Stay out of spaces you know to be contaminated to the extent possible or spend as little time as possible there. Open a window if you can. See if you can work at home at least part of the time if your work environment is toxic. Modify your cosmetics requirements—can you live without that manicure or perm?

When you travel, bring your own personal care products with you. If you have wisely selected toothpaste, mouthwash, soap, shampoo, and conditioner made with plant oils and other recognizable natural substances, why settle for chemical-laden alternatives at a hotel?

Another entire book would be needed to adequately address the issue of cleaning up commercial indoor spaces. Do some research on your own and band with others to begin to address and remedy the situation.

The Story Condensed

Your personal care products, cosmetics, household cleaners, laundry soap, and many other everyday products may be chock full of dozens of chemicals that are inflammators and hormone disrupters. These chemicals usually get into your body after being absorbed by your skin or your lungs. When buying such items, keep the following guidelines in mind.

- Manufacturers face few restrictions in formulating these products. Just because you can buy something in the supermarket, drugstore, or even a natural products store doesn't mean it is free of potentially harmful ingredients.
- The long-term consequence to people of the vast majority of manmade chemicals in personal care and household

products is not known. Testing on animals is useless and misleading. Use your shopping dollars to opt out of testing these chemicals on your own body.

- If a personal care or cleaning product has chemicals with long names or any sort of artificial fragrance, shop until you find a product with recognizable ingredients. Choose products that are either fragrance free or scented only with natural plant oils.

- Read ingredients in the fine print, not prominent label endorsements such as "natural" or "physician recommended." Such label wording is unregulated and largely meaningless. Check Chapter 21, *Perfect Resources,* for sites where you can get more information on product ingredients.

- Make simpler choices, such as using fewer personal care products and using glass or stainless steel cookware instead of pots with artificial coating. If you travel, bring your own personal care products with you.

- You may need to buy many of your personal care products and cosmetics in "health food" stores or on the Internet. You can get cleaning products from the same sources, or learn to make your own with such basic ingredients as baking soda, vinegar, and lemon juice. Ideas abound online.

- Before infrequent household purchases, from sheets and paint to pots and carpets, take the time to go to credible, independent sources to learn which choices are the friendliest to the environment and your health. Information is available in your library and on many good Internet sites. Beware that industry-funded sites or organizations may have consumer friendly names. If a source tells you there's no health threat from industrial chemicals, find a more balanced opinion.

- Being healthy and looking good are inseparable. You won't be attractive for long if your skin, hair, nails, and cells are harmed by toxic chemicals.

Choosing truly natural and nontoxic personal care and cleaning products goes hand-in-hand with the Perfect Formula Diet. Once you're on a Perfect Foods eating plan, detoxifying household products can be your next step up in freeing yourself from inflammators, losing weight, reinforcing health, and looking good. And remember, Perfect Foods have substances that support and speed the process of detoxifying from past exposure to harmful chemicals.

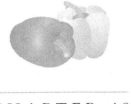

CHAPTER 18

Perfect Next Steps

The Perfect Formula Diet is the foundation for attaining the health and weight you always wanted. You can't make up for poor food choices through any other lifestyle measure, including exercise, sleep, or meditation.

The ideas in this chapter complement, rather than replace, the Perfect Formula Diet. As you feel better, it's natural to raise the bar in more aspects of your life. Luckily for you, the choice between healthy eating and other positive life choices is not either-or. In fact, feeling great through eating Perfect Foods will encourage you to make other desirable changes in your everyday routines.

You Are Designed To Move

Even if you shun exercise, your naturally Perfect Body wants to move. A sedentary lifestyle is unnatural, while physical conditioning can have a significant impact on balancing your body's pro- and anti-inflammatory forces.

Multiple studies have found that more physical activity results in lower CRP levels. People who exercise tend to live longer and are less likely to be disabled. However, weight trumps exercise in determining levels of chronic inflammation.

Active muscles function as the largest organ in your body, working as an integral part of your endocrine, immune, and nervous systems. Contracting your muscles will substantially, but temporarily, increase your body's level of IL-6. During physical activity, IL-6 stimulates the liver to release more glucose to burn and also increases the body's ability to burn fat for fuel.

Previous chapters on health explain that while IL-6 is generally regarded as a sign of inflammation, pro-inflammatory substances are also one trigger for the release of anti-inflammatory substances. Those who exercise more actually have a lower *resting* IL-6 level, which indicates a reduced level of chronic inflammation.

In the case of exercise, the net effect of contracting muscle appears to help balance pro- and anti-inflammatory forces and increase your body's ability to deal with other inflammators by strengthening immunity. However, exercise that is too intense or prolonged can lower immunity.

In addition to its benefits in balancing inflammation, physical activity strengthens your heart muscle itself and reduces the tendency of blood to clot. In fact, you need exercise for healthy muscle growth. Using your muscles destroys old and dysfunctional muscle cells so stronger and larger new cells will grow.

Workouts can also trigger the release of your body's endorphins, "feel good" substances that reward your decision to move. Weight-bearing activity strengthens your bones as well as your muscles. Movement burns calories, which helps you get to your Perfect Weight faster—but you already knew that!

You can easily learn more about the various types of exercise and which are best for your current state of fitness and interests. *If you're not already in excellent shape, or if you have any chronic illness, make your doctor your first stop so you can understand what level of exercise is safe to start out with and how fast you can reasonably progress.*

Consider hiring a personal trainer for a fast start to a conditioning program. More economically, try public recreation centers, library books, or reliable websites for advice and information.

Find an enjoyable activity you can do with a friend and make physical activity part of your daily routine. Moving your body can be convenient, inexpensive, fun, and rewarding, so there's no reason to put off your fitness plan.

Sleep: Effortless Healing

While exercise may seem daunting, sleeping is totally effortless. If you have insomnia, falling and staying asleep may be a challenge, but sleep itself is simple enough for the youngest baby to master.

Sleep is an active biological state that underlies good physical and mental health, affecting mood and the functioning of the nervous, endocrine, and immune systems. For all warm-blooded animals, sleep is necessary for survival.

From the standpoint of scientific understanding, sleep is the most mysterious body function. Despite decades of expensive research and brutalizing countless animals in labs, scientists still have no clear understanding of the functions or mechanisms of sleep.

The pro- and anti-inflammatory balance in your body fluctuates naturally over the course of each 24-hour period. Inflammation is generally higher at night, worsening chronic conditions such as asthma.

Scientists can observe what happens to people who are sleep-deprived. One of the most obvious effects is sleepiness—the body wants what it needs to survive, and sleep is a necessity.

Sleep-deprivation, both short term and long term, is an inflammator. Multiple studies find that inflammatory markers rise after sleep loss or disturbance, increasing general pain and fatigue as well as the risk of chronic inflammatory illness, including cardiovascular disease, arthritis, and diabetes. Another study found that one night of sleep loss stimulated both pro- and anti-inflammatory processes. Other researchers have concluded that the number of immune cells rises after sleep deprivation, but these cells don't work very well and aren't effective.

Sleep patterns translate into disease risk. Some studies have found that people who sleep seven to eight hours a night generally have the lowest risk of developing chronic illnesses such as diabetes, coronary disease, and high blood pressure and have the lowest overall chance of dying. Other studies have found that six to seven hours of sleep a night is the most beneficial for health. In any case, too much sleep is no better than too little.

A fascinating study in Sweden examined 20 years of records to link the number of heart attacks to changes from daylight savings time to standard time and back again. When clocks were set back an hour on Sunday (standard time), there were measurably fewer heart attacks than normal on Monday as people benefited from an extra hour of sleep.

On the Monday through Wednesday following the change to daylight saving time and the loss of an hour of sleep, researchers observed up to a 10% increase in the number of heart attacks. This study vividly demonstrates key links among sleep, inflammation, and health outcomes.

Sleep also affects body weight. Not getting sufficient sleep can foster increased appetite, lower insulin sensitivity, and weight gain.

The quality of your sleep and the ease of falling and staying asleep may improve on the Perfect Formula Diet—this result needs more study. The normalization of hormones and pro- and anti-inflammatory forces on this whole foods eating plan may have a beneficial effect, leading to natural sleep at night and less sleepiness and fatigue during the day. An active inflammatory process may underlie at least some sleep disruption.

The clear message is to get the amount of sleep your Perfect Body wants without artificial manipulations of either stimulants or sleeping pills. This will likely be six to eight hours a night. Most adults who are sleep deprived select a late bedtime because they're staying up late to get work done, watch television, or use the Internet.

The bottom line is that delaying going to bed can be a difficult habit to break, but is definitely your choice. Calling it a night at a time that allows for seven to eight hours of sleep may be your next step up after you begin the Perfect Formula Diet.

Stress And Emotion: The Soft Factors In Your Health
Because your brain and nervous system are so closely linked to hormone levels, inflammation, and immune system functioning, the stress and emotions you experience will impact your health. These "soft" factors are difficult to measure and study; nonetheless, researchers have started to gauge the impact. Here are some examples.

- Stress can raise cholesterol levels.
- Stress can deplete neurotransmitters, possibly leading to depression.
- Unpleasant emotions and stress can trigger inflammation and interfere with immune system functioning.
- Prolonged job stress resulting in a state of burn-out increases systemic inflammation and raises cardiovascular risk.
- Loneliness and isolation raise the risk of death and illness from two to five times, regardless of other health-impacting choices. Quality of relationships is more important than quantity.
- Stress can aggravate many conditions based on chronic inflammation, including gum disease, some autoimmune illnesses, arthritis, migraines, and asthma.

Helpful and effective strategies to manage stress, such as yoga, meditation, and guided imagery, can brighten your outlook and improve body metabolism. Enjoyable music also helps blood vessels function better and can help offset the harmful effects of stress.

Consult a professional for counseling if you have difficulties managing stress on your own. Personal contact with a counselor, coach, or support group can also be beneficial in maintaining weight loss.

Green Spaces: Where People Were Meant To Be
A few pioneering studies show that your health can benefit from spending time in or even just looking at green space, which is open,

undeveloped land with trees and other plants. This effect is not due to increased exercise while you are in a park.

Time spent in green spaces translates to fewer deaths from cardiovascular disease and all causes combined as well as simply feeling healthier. Being in nature helps overcome stress and fatigue and may reduce feelings of anger, frustration, and aggression.

While scientists don't understand why natural settings are so beneficial, don't let that stop you from taking advantage of this effect. Put pictures of beautiful natural places in your home and work space, take advantage of green views, and spend as much time outdoors in nature as you can. Work with others to protect green and wild places so you'll always have this refuge.

Smoking And Drugs: Don't

If you still use tobacco, you know how dangerous this is. Smoking causes inflammation and health problems throughout your body and raises CRP levels. Decide to quit, and do it! You have limitless resources to help you out.

Eating the Perfect Formula Diet while you smoke is like taking aspirin for a headache while you continue to bang your head against a wall. Ditto for taking illegal drugs, over-imbibing in alcohol, and abusing prescription drugs. All these assaults on your Perfect Body undermine many of the beneficial effects of a whole-food eating plan.

Use the Perfect Formula Diet as a reason to get the help you need and turn your life around. You can enhance your well-being to the point that artificial "feel good" boosters become truly second-rate and unappealing.

How Did Humans Survive All This Time?

Does it seem natural that you would need drugs for your body to accomplish the most basic functions necessary for survival?

- Breathing
- Digesting food

- Sleeping
- Urinating
- Eliminating
- Nerve functioning
- Heart beating in proper rhythm and with sufficient force
- Blood chemistry maintenance
- Blood sugar maintenance

Certainly the design of your naturally Perfect Body couldn't be that deficient. Otherwise, humans would never have been able to survive and reproduce over the centuries before medications were manufactured.

Wild animals, able to select the food best suited for their species and to live and sleep as nature designed, are able to carry out these basic functions without drugs or surgery.

Whatever lifestyle choices are compromising your body's ability to carry out basic functions can be altered. With that change, your health could then improve because the *fundamental cause* of illness would be reduced or eliminated.

Taking drugs to get healthy is like using credit card A (with 16% interest) to pay off credit card B (with 18% interest). You may be better off—or you might not be, if there are hidden zingers in the fine print of credit card A. In either case, this strategy is not likely to get you out of debt.

To continue the analogy, drugs may improve your health—unless the side effects turn out to be worse than your original disease. However, drugs are no more likely to cure or reverse your chronic illness than using credit card A is to result in a debt-free, financially sound status for you.

Just What Are The Side-Effects?
In 2005, more than 15,000 people died from side effects of prescription medications and almost 90,000 reactions serious enough to be reported to the FDA occurred.

As a next step after you get started on the Perfect Formula Diet, you might choose to research the potential side effects of any medications you're taking. Keep notes of your findings to discuss with your physician. Just as doctors were slow to acknowledge the dangers of tobacco use, so many physicians may not immediately recognize side effects you may be suffering from your medications. You may need to shop around for a physician who is open to treatment methods that go beyond drugs.

Publication bias in the journals your doctor respects may be at least partially responsible for this dangerous state. In a major study, researchers tracked journal articles on every prescription drug approved by the Food and Drug Administration (FDA) from 1998 to 2000. The researchers conclude that studies showing a drug was effective were substantially more likely to be published than studies showing a drug didn't work or had side effects. This lack of convenient access to complete information impacts doctors' abilities to be totally informed.

With medical supervision and agreement, you may be able to cut down or eliminate prescription and nonprescription medications once you are consistently following the Perfect Formula Diet. Never change the dose or timing of or eliminate a medication without your physician's assent and guidance.

Alternative Medicine: Another Effective Partner

If drugs and surgery lose their luster as first-choice means to deal with illness, you might consider whether alternative therapies could help any symptoms that remain after you get onto the Perfect Formula Diet and follow the major next steps (exercise, sleep, coping with stress, seeking green spaces, stopping smoking and substance abuse, and minimizing potentially toxic chemicals in your environment).

Alternative methods, which can be preventive as well as curative, include acupuncture, chiropractic, herbs, and mind-body therapies (guided imagery, yoga, biofeedback, meditation, and many others).

As discussed earlier in this book, mega-doses of vitamins and minerals are more likely to be harmful than helpful, so pursue this course *only* if prescribed by your doctor for a specific *diagnosed* medical condition (for example, anemia).

Alternative medicine can be effective and cost less than conventional medical treatment. However, the mechanisms of action of most alternative therapies are not well understood.

For example, acupuncture may reduce chronic inflammation through its effect on the nervous system, and other alternative methods may also dampen chronic inflammation. Acupuncture may also strengthen the immune system and can be effective for treatment of cardiovascular disease, high blood pressure, congestive heart failure, and pain.

Mind-body techniques may work through the influence that the brain has on the functioning of the immune, endocrine, and nervous systems. These techniques may reduce recovery time after surgery, mitigate pain for a range of conditions, and improve coping and quality of life. For example, a study of 225 overweight women found that those who received intensive relaxation response training had less psychological stress and medical symptoms over a two year period and didn't gain any weight during this time.

Seek help from a licensed professional, if possible, in considering alternative treatments. If practitioners are not licensed in the modality you're interested in, carefully check the training and credentials of any person from whom you seek advice or care. Also thoroughly research online or use other information sources to be sure the practitioner and approach are reputable; then share your use of alternative modalities with your physician.

The Story Condensed

Once you adopt the Perfect Formula Diet and start weighing less and feeling better, you may want to take further steps to improve your health and decrease chronic inflammation. However, if you make changes in other areas without the dietary underpinnings, the long-term effects on your health and weight will most likely be marginal.

The chapters *Perfect Planet* and *Perfect Home* describe how critical it is to get as many potentially toxic chemicals as possible out of your life and out of your Perfect Body. The steps below are best taken at the same time as or after this detoxifying action program.

- Exercise: Start a regular conditioning program and ramp up your fitness level to enjoy the balancing effects of movement on inflammation and the overall beneficial impact on many other aspects of your health; be sure to get supervision and input from your health care professional as appropriate.
- Sleep: Get the amount of sleep your naturally Perfect Body wants when you don't use stimulants or sleeping pills; benefits may include reduced chronic inflammation and higher energy levels during the day.
- Stress: Cultivate helpful coping mechanisms, develop high quality relationships with others, and seek counseling if needed.
- Green spaces: Spend as much time as you can in beautiful outdoor settings and protect these settings as a refuge for health.
- Smoking and illegal drugs: Get the help you need to stop using tobacco as well as illegal substances that your naturally Perfect Body is not designed to handle.
- Prescription and over-the-counter drugs: Research side effects, discuss with your doctor, and see if you can reduce or eliminate use of these drugs as you benefit from the Perfect Formula Diet and other next steps; *never change the dose or discontinue use of any medication without your physician's oversight and consent.*
- Alternative medicine: Consider whether acupuncture, herbs, guided imagery, or other alternative treatments are right for you; *be sure to seek out reputable professionals and information sources to help you and let your physician know about your use of these treatments.*

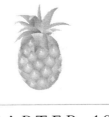

CHAPTER 19

Perfect Climate

Imagine you're in the area of your workplace where people casually gather, maybe a kitchen, break room, or lunch room. One of your co-workers just celebrated a birthday, and a large wedge of your favorite chocolate cake is left out for the taking. You've decided to follow the Perfect Formula Diet and know the cake was made with milk and eggs. But at the same time, you're so tempted. After a struggling hesitation, you may or may not devour the cake. Either way, you feel trapped with a lose-lose decision.

Now imagine that, instead of cake, you found a co-worker's purse in the same room. You notice the purse is open and a $50 bill is partly sticking out. You know whose purse it is—a new employee with two kids to support. You have not met her, but have heard she is just getting back to work after a long and difficult period of unemployment.

How tempted are you to pocket the $50? If you are like most people, that idea may be a fleeting thought which never has much appeal. In fact, you are probably repelled by the idea. You snatch the purse and take off to return it to its rightful owner. After, you feel great about yourself and relieved at the happy ending.

When will you consistently and effortlessly stick to the Perfect Formula Diet? When you see eating the chocolate cake as unacceptable

229

as stealing the $50. You can get to that point with just a little bit of knowledge and empathy.

Your commitment is vital to succeeding on a Perfect Foods eating plan. Ironically, the promise of better health and weight loss, as well as good intentions, may be insufficient incentive to eat healthy all the time. When you consider *all* the reasons you should stick to the Perfect Formula Diet, you stabilize your motivation, just as having several legs steadies a chair. *To dependably stay on the healthiest diet, with no lapses, you will benefit from moral reasons and ethical purpose outside yourself.*

Protecting our planet to create a sustainable future for yourself and the young people you care about can be one foundation of your inspiration. This chapter reinforces your commitment to your health and to Perfect Foods. *Stoke your motivation by understanding that raising and catching animals (including fish) for food are major contributors to global warming and to our dangerous degradation of farmlands, ecosystems, air, and water.*

Extreme Weather And You

If you live on planet earth, you would be well advised to place mitigating climate change on the top of your list of priorities. While the weather was at one time a subject for superficial chit-chat, now serious conversations about climate rank with any critical topic for discussion.

The term "global warming," although commonly used, is not sufficiently descriptive of the changes sweeping worldwide climate patterns. "Climate destabilization" is a more accurate, vivid indicator of what scientists are observing.

Some media stories, in the service of special interests, deny that climate destabilization is related to human activities, or even that it's happening at all. However, the worldwide consensus of respected researchers is that the planetary climate is undergoing rapid, significant change fueled by human activities that accumulate heat-trapping greenhouse gases.

It's Happening Now And It's Hurting You

Climate destabilization is wreaking havoc already, and not waiting for a distant future. Stop and think about how life-changing this is. These problems, which you've seen again and again in heart-wrenching news stories, will only intensify over time:

- Changes in rain and snowfall patterns, resulting in droughts, flooding, and shortages of fresh water
- More severe and frequent rain storms, windstorms, torna-does, and hurricanes
- Extremes of temperature compared to what people have historically seen around the world, with more frequent and hotter heat waves and also increased cold waves
- More intense, larger, and numerous wildfires, resulting in the destruction of natural resources and lost homes
- Warmer and more acidic, oxygen-poor ocean water that kills billions of sea creatures and plants and destroys coral reefs
- Far-reaching extinction of the animals and plants forming the web of life on our planet
- Spread of tree-killing beetles that are devastating tens of millions of acres of healthy forests
- Redistribution of the weight of ice and ocean water on the earth's crust, resulting in more volcanic eruptions, tsunamis, and earthquakes
- Melting glaciers, coastal erosion, and flooding

The financial consequences *will* overshadow any banking or housing cost meltdown:

- Escalating human poverty around the world and hundreds of millions of climate refugees
- Lost and failed crops, resulting in higher food prices and eventually food shortages

- National and local economic stress from the cost of dealing with ever more numerous and devastating natural disasters

Maybe you, a loved one, or a friend has already experienced natural disaster from climate destabilization. Dreams and lives were shattered by tornadoes, a house burned to the ground, disastrous flooding, or jobs lost from damaged workplaces.

Even the staid insurance industry, hardly a bastion of radical thought, recognizes the severe threat and is grappling with how to deal with it. One solution for these companies is to abandon selling policies in high-risk areas, leaving taxpayers to foot the entire bill for weather-related damage.

The time to act is **now** *and you have an indispensable contribution to make. The Perfect Formula Diet, the healthiest choice for you, also slams the brakes on climate destabilization.*

Your Health Suffers Directly

Climate destabilization is a direct threat to human health worldwide. Doctors, the World Health Organization, and other public health officials raise the red flag.

- Warmer weather fuels outbreaks of infectious and insect-borne diseases including West Nile virus, encephalitis, dengue fever, malaria, and cholera, not to mention death from heat stroke.
- For the period 1970 to 2004, heat and drought killed more Americans than any other category of natural disaster.
- Water-borne illnesses spread more easily and people may be forced to use polluted water for drinking and bathing.
- People drown in floods, die in wildfires, and are exposed to the elements after losing their homes.
- Pollen season begins earlier and explodes with more pollen, hurting those with allergies and asthma.
- Crop failures and higher food prices directly lead to food riots, malnutrition, and even starvation.

- The effects of climate destabilization threaten security and prosperity and motivate wars over scarce resources.

Farming Animals: A Planetary Threat

Here's some excellent news. If everyone in the world went on an animal-free diet, the reduction in climate destabilization would be greater than if every car, truck, train, ship, and airplane were sidelined. The United Nation report *Livestock's Long Shadow* concludes that while transportation releases 16% of all greenhouse gas emissions around the world, farming animals to eat generates 18% of greenhouse gases.

Raising animals for food produces two potent greenhouse gases, methane and nitrous oxide. Molecule for molecule, methane warms the planet 24 times more powerfully than carbon dioxide. Nitrous oxide is even more dangerous, with 320 times the power to destabilize climate compared to carbon dioxide.

University of Chicago researchers reinforce the UN report. If you eat a typical amount of meat, you're responsible for releasing one and a half tons more greenhouse gases every year than someone on an animal-free diet. Fish is almost as destructive as meat in its effect on climate because of the fuel used by fishing boats and the resources needed for "fish farms."

A German study concluded that a meat-based diet would—every single year—release the greenhouse gas equivalent of driving almost 3,000 miles in a mid-size car. In contrast, the "carbon footprint" of a plant-based diet would be equivalent to only about 390 miles of driving and an organic plant-based diet to 175 miles.

While "eating locally" is a worthy goal, the impact of choosing food from close-by sources will be of small value in helping the climate if the foods you buy or raise are meat and dairy. How food is produced and processed determines 83% of that food's impact on global warming, while how far it is transported has much less significance.

You can choose to emulate the millions who have already found a healthier and less damaging way to eat by sticking to plants. If we band together in this endeavor, we can have an *immediate* impact on the future of the planet. Your choice is the place where you start, so don't underestimate the power of your actions.

Digging Deeper

Why is raising animals for food so damaging to the climate and to earth's life support systems? To understand, you need to follow the end-to-end process of producing animal foods.

When you look at meat, dairy foods, and eggs what you don't immediately see is all the food the animal needed to make the muscle, mammary secretions, and reproductive materials you're about to eat. At least two to three pounds of feed are needed to produce a pound of chicken, four to six pounds of feed for a pound of pork, and seven to ten pounds of feed for a pound of beef. Thirty nine calories of plant food are needed to produce one calorie from an egg.

Growing this animal feed uses fertilizers, herbicides, and pesticides—usually made from petrochemicals in processes that produce their own greenhouse gases—and land. Irrigating feed crops and operating farm machinery both require energy that generates even more greenhouse gases.

To clear room to grow more and more feed for more and more farmed animals, people are chopping down and burning forests at an accelerating rate. The loss of these forests is one of the major contributors to climate destabilization, as forests store so much carbon. Cattle ranches are destroying the Amazon rainforest. People also drain wetlands to grow animal feed, which releases all the carbon dioxide trapped in the wetlands soil.

Food animals live on huge factory farms in most parts of the world. Their manure, untreated, is stored in huge "lagoons" near the farms, emitting the powerful greenhouse gases nitrous oxide and methane.

Once they're deemed large enough to eat, animals are transported to slaughterhouses, killed, "processed," refrigerated, transported to stores, and cooked, all of which also require energy and produce greenhouse gases.

Cows, goats, and sheep all directly emit methane produced in their digestive tracts at both ends of the animals. Dairy cows produce more methane per animal than do cows raised solely for meat.

Green As Far As You Can See And Imagine

Your children and grandchildren will need food, fresh and clean water, breathable air, topsoil, land, forests, energy, and other vital resources to survive. You will also require these basics for life, which you may be taking too much for granted.

In 2006, it took our planet 15 months to regenerate the natural resources used in 12 months—clearly not a sustainable situation. The pace of depletion grows more unsupportable each year. *By 2050, scientists estimate it would take two planet earths to provide the natural resources people expect; this would increase to three planets if everyone had the animal-based eating habits of those in developed countries.*

Raising animals for food is a massive cause of resource consumption, land degradation, air pollution, water pollution, water shortages, and loss of biodiversity. Accounting for land needed to raise feed and for grazing, farmed animals use 70% of all agricultural land and 30% of the land surface of our planet. Topsoil is eroding 30 times faster than it is forming and the remaining soil is stripped of key nutrients.

The process of raising farmed animals produces almost two thirds of the ammonia emitted into the atmosphere, causing acid rain and more destruction of ecosystems.

Feeding animals to produce human food is wasteful and inefficient. Growing soybeans, rice, or corn coaxes more than 200 pounds of protein per acre from the soil, while meat averages only 45 pounds of protein per acre. You could grow 145 pounds of potatoes with the same fossil fuel needed to produce one pound of beef.

Just as staggering, you could grow 200 pounds of potatoes with the same water required for that pound of beef. Overall, producing a meat-based diet uses more than 4,000 gallons of water each day for just one person, but a plant-based diet requires only 300 gallons a day of this precious resource. *With climate destabilization causing more droughts, a water-conserving plant-based diet becomes even more critical.*

Agriculture, much of it aimed at raising animal feed, uses 85% of U.S. freshwater consumption every year. Farmed animals cause water pollution through feces and urine, antibiotics and hormones fed to them to make them grow faster, runoff from fertilizers and pesticides used to grow feed, and erosion from overgrazing and trampling the earth.

You might have heard that processing grain into biofuel is driving up food prices and destroying habitat as more land is farmed. However, more than seven times more grain is fed to farmed animals each year than is turned into biofuel. Animals eat about 40% of all grain grown worldwide, wasting 50% to 90% of the grain's energy in the process.

What You Gain

Don't miss this soul-satisfying opportunity to substantially help yourself and everyone around you simply by making a change in eating habits. What you choose to do does matter. Just as Perfect Foods nourish your body, purpose nourishes your soul.

*Being "green" is not an optional nice thing to do. Your life and the next generation need you to start conserving **now** for a sustainable future. Boosting your health and sculpting your weight with the Perfect Formula Diet is a great gift in so many ways—to yourself and to everyone you care about. An animal-free diet is socially desirable and praiseworthy.*

Advocating for collective action is critical. But if you wait for governments worldwide to get their act together before you take action, climate destabilization will just keep accelerating.

Many Motivations, Same Result

Maybe climate destabilization is not a cause that grabs you emotionally. For purposes of sticking to the Perfect Formula Diet, this is okay. You can choose from any compelling ethical reason to choose Perfect Foods and shun other foods.

- Saving children. According to the United Nations Children's Fund, more than 5,000,000 children die every year from inadequate nutrition. When you stop eating animal foods, the feed set aside for cows, chickens, farmed fish, and other creatures can now go to nourish these children.
- Compassion for animals—spare the "farmed" animals a short, painful, unnatural life, separation at birth from their babies, and an agonizing death just so their bodies and secretions will provide you with illness-producing fat and protein.
- Spiritual reasons—once you start choosing a plant-only diet, you will effortlessly evolve spiritually to feel closer to nature, animals, and the divinity in the universe, however you believe that to manifest. While you are eating animal foods, this spiritual evolution is a grueling struggle.

Let your passion guide you in discovering compelling reasons to stick to the Perfect Formula Diet. You can relate just about anything you care about back to your health, energy level, compassion, empathy, ethics, and desire for a better future.

Join the evolution to a whole-foods, plant-based diet, just as many well-known figures already have. Here is a sampling from happycow.net, an excellent site that tracks animal-free diets, of celebrities thriving on plant-based eating.

- Actors: including Ellen DeGeneres, Woody Harrelson, Eric Roberts, Daryl Hannah, Alicia Silverstone, Linda Blair, Kevin Nealon, and James Cromwell
- Singers: including Moby, Nellie McKay, Fiona Apple, Erykah Badu, Jason Mraz, Alanis Morissette, and Chrissie Hynde
- Other public figures: including Coretta Scott King, Dan Piraro, and Dr. Benjamin Spock

The Story Condensed

Raising animals for food is a massive force intensifying climate destabilization and all its catastrophic effects. You make the difference and reduce your carbon footprint when you choose the Perfect Formula Diet.

Instead of "seafood," "see" your food for what it is, so you can contribute to a green, sustainable future for yourself and everyone you care about. See stick-thin children lying listlessly in their desperate mothers' arms, cows hung by their hind legs to suffer prolonged and agonizing deaths, and fish writhing in pain and struggling for a last molecule of oxygen.

Look at meat and see polar bears drowning as their icy homes melt. Look at dairy products and see drought-driven wildfires hot enough to melt street signs—and people's dreams. Look at fish and see vanishing penguins, butchered dolphins, and empty oceans. Look at eggs and see Hurricane Katrina victims huddled in the Superdome, grieving over their lost families. Then, you can stick to a healthy diet for yourself with no hesitations or lapses.

See food, see it for what it *really* embodies, and permanently transform your weight and your health.

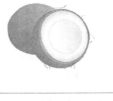

CHAPTER 20

Perfect Story

This book tells the tale of Perfect Foods and their profound positive significance for your weight and health. As a quick reference, this chapter summarizes the highlights of the story of the Perfect Formula Diet.

- Your naturally Perfect Body will stay lean and healthy—without hunger or portion control—as soon as you get out of your own way. Eat the foods you're designed for and avoid toxic chemicals drenching your environment.
- Your overall *pattern* of eating is the most important choice determining your weight and health. Marginal dietary changes—one apple or some other "super food" a day—will yield insignificant improvement.
- Perfect Foods include colorful vegetables, yummy fruits, satisfying potatoes and beans, filling whole grains, aromatic herbs and spices, and crunchy nuts and seeds.
- You get the ideal amount of protein from Perfect Foods because plants put together *all* the essential amino acids in your body. "Animal protein" doesn't have any extra ingredients missing from plant protein. In fact, animal protein is simply recycled plant protein.

- On the Perfect Formula Diet, by volume, one quarter of your food is vegetables, one quarter fruit, one quarter a mixture of beans and potatoes, and one quarter whole grains. Prepare your foods to be flavorful with abundant herbs and spices. Add a handful of nuts or seeds four to six times a week.
- Eat when you are moderately hungry and stop when you're full. Don't worry about "meals." Over time you will discover the "not-meal" plans that work for you.
- Your commitment to the Perfect Formula Diet will grow as your health and vigor soar and your body sculpts itself. Effective food-planning strategies will get you started and accelerate your momentum.
- If you live in a developed country, you'll probably die from a disease aggravated by chronic inflammation, which may be provoked by foreign proteins in your food. Insulin-like growth hormone-1 (IGF-1), estrogen and other hormones in meat and dairy foods, and toxic molecules formed in cooking may also contribute significantly to your health problems.
- Next steps to reinforce the happy Perfect Formula Diet results include getting toxic chemicals out of your home and personal care products, exercise, optimal sleep, and spending time in green places.
- Our planet cannot provide the resources to support billions of people eating meat, fish, animal milk, and eggs indefinitely. The shrinking natural resources we have now are degraded and squandered when people use animals for food.
- Farming animals for food contributes mightily to climate destabilization, pollution, and water shortages *now,* not in some mythical distant future. The Perfect Formula Diet heals the earth along with you. Stay committed to your eating choices for the right reasons—all the reasons—and you're certain to be successful!

Your challenge now is to decide what to do with this profoundly transformative knowledge. Will you join the swelling ranks of fellow citizens discovering that a plant-based, whole-foods diet is delicious, appealing, and the overall best choice? Will you slim to your desired weight, invigorate your health, and shake up your life? Your naturally Perfect Body is cheering for you.

CHAPTER 21

Perfect Resources

With millions of people on the journey to a whole-foods diet, chemical-free personal care and cleaning products, and healthy, fulfilling life choices, you're sure to find the information and support you need for your success. This section will help you discover a wealth of resources to ease the way and build your commitment.

Have fun searching out your own favorites. It's a great way to stay balanced on the surfboard and move forward.

Note that some recipes in the sources below call for manufactured oils, white flour, or other less-than-perfect foods. As you become a more skilled cook, you'll learn to leave out the less healthy ingredients or substitute healthier ones (such as whole wheat pasta for white pasta or brown rice for white rice). If you are not used to the taste of whole grains, you can transition painlessly by starting out mixing whole grains and refined grains half and half, and then gradually increasing the proportion of whole grains.

One great technique, described in detail by Dr. John and Mary McDougall, is to sauté food in small amounts of water, vegetable broth, wine, or juice instead of oil. The results taste spectacular and your Perfect Body will respond to the vastly improved food as weight melts away. See any of the Dr. McDougall resources for more information.

Perfect Food Recipes–Online

Excellent—you are guaranteed to find delicious recipes on this superb site

http://www.fatfreevegan.com

Dr. McDougall Newsletter—every edition has fantastic recipes! Mary McDougall is a cooking genius who has lovingly crafted thousands of delicious, satisfying, easy-to-make recipes using low-cost ingredients. Never settle for a dull not-meal.

Here are some issues to get you started. November 2007 and December 2007 have collections of one-pot and easy-to-prepare family favorites. February 2008 presents more favorites, some a bit more geared to special meals with guests. March 2008 features recipes for the frugal cook.

www.drmcdougall.com/newsletter/archive.html

Lots more great ideas

www.nutritionmd.org/index.html
www.vrg.org/recipes/index.htm
www.vegweb.com
http://veganchef.com

Perfect Food Recipes–Books

Fat-Free & Easy; The Peaceful Palate, both by Jennifer Raymond

Vegetarian Soups for All Seasons; Vegan Express, both by Nava Atlas

The McDougall Quick & Easy Cookbook, John McDougall, M.D. and Mary McDougall

The Engine 2 Diet, Rip Esselstyn (excellent recipes in last part of this book)

Fabulous Beans, Barb Bloomfield

Vegan Vittles, Joanne Stepaniak

How to Eat Like a Vegetarian Even if You Never Want to Be One,
Carol J. Adams and Patti Breitman

The Best in the World, Neal Barnard, M.D.

The Best in the World II, Jennifer Keller, R.D.

Vegan Planet, Robin Robertson

Where To Buy Perfect Foods

Your local supermarket is sure to have a colorful aisle of fruits and vegetables, dairy-free milks, frozen or refrigerated meat substitutes, dried beans, and lots of other Perfect Foods. However, you'll be amazed at the choices of fresh and prepared Perfect Foods in natural foods stores. *Search the Internet to locate chains or individual stores near you.* Note: stores with mostly supplements are NOT natural foods stores.

Natural foods stores are also the most convenient place to buy personal care and cleaning products that are free of harmful chemicals. However, even if you buy food or household products at a natural foods store, you still need to read the label. Not everything in a natural foods store is a Perfect Food or free of harmful chemicals.

The largest chain of natural foods stores is Whole Foods. Find your closest location at *http://www.wholefoodsmarket.com.* You can check whether you live near a Trader Joe's at *http://traderjoes.com.* This chain has a unique and ever-changing selection of Perfect Foods and nontoxic cleaners, often at lower prices than other natural foods stores.

Find a natural foods cooperative near you, *www.coopdirectory.org/directory.htm.*

Farmers markets support small, local growers and are the ideal source for Perfect Foods. Simply enter "farmers market" and the name of your community into any good Internet search engine to see your tasty options.

If you don't live near a natural foods or farmers market, type whatever you're looking for into any good search engine and buy it online. Here are a few ideas.

http://www.drfuhrman.com/shop/healthy_additions.aspx A new, innovative food line from Dr. Fuhrman.

www.rightfoods.com Dr. McDougall's line of healthy convenience foods. Find hot water and eat healthy anywhere.

http://www.healthy-eating.com

http://veganessentials.com See the food tab.

www.chocolatedecadence.com Now this is REAL chocolate.

Marine Algae Omega-3 Fatty Acids

Several brands are available to supply long chain omega-3 fatty acids directly from marine algae, bypassing the toxic chemicals and environmental devastation of fish oil.

Examples include Deva Vegan Omega-3 DHA (order at *www.devanutrition.com*), Dr. Fuhrman's DHA Purity (order at *http://www.drfuhrman.com/shop/DHA.aspx*), and NuTru O-Mega-Zen3 (order at *http://nutru.com*). Be careful that the supplement is animal-free. *Read the label ingredients carefully.*

Websites On Health, Weight, And Nutrition

www.pcrm.org
www.drmcdougall.com
http://drgreger.org
www.drfuhrman.com
www.diseaseproof.com
www.ruthheidrich.com
www.jeffnovick.com
www.vrg.org
www.vegsource.com
http://thechinastudy.com

www.notmilk.com
http://atkinsdietalert.org
http://atkinsexposed.org
www.compassionatecooks.com
www.theengine2diet.com
www.exsalus.com
www.ravediet.com
www.plantbasednutrition.org

Books On Health, Weight, And Nutrition

The China Study, T. Colin Campbell, Ph.D.

Breaking the Food Seduction; Dr. Neal Barnard's Program for Reversing Diabetes; Foods that Fight Pain; A Physician's Slimming Guide for Permanent Weight Control; Turn off the Fat Genes; Food for Life, all by Neal Barnard, M.D.

The McDougall Program for Women; Digestive Tune-Up; The McDougall Program for Maximum Weight Loss; The McDougall Program for a Healthy Heart, all by John McDougall, M.D.

Eat to Live, Joel Fuhrman, M.D.

Becoming Vegan: The Complete Guide to Adopting a Healthy Plant-Based Diet, Brenda Davis and Vesanto Melina

Eat More, Weigh Less, Dean Ornish, M.D.

Skinny Bitch, Rory Freedman and Kim Barnouin

Carbophobia: The Sorry Truth About America's Low-Carb Craze; Bird Flu: A Virus of Our Own Hatching, both by Michael Greger, M.D.

The Food Revolution, John Robbins

The Pleasure Trap, Douglas Lisle

Prevent and Reverse Heart Disease, Caldwell B. Esselstyn, M.D.

A Race for Life; CHEF; Senior Fitness, all by Ruth Heidrich, Ph.D.

The Engine 2 Diet, Rip Esselstyn

Healthy Eating for Life for Children, PCRM with Amy Lanou, Ph.D.

Healthy Eating for Life for Women, PCRM with Kristine Kieswer

Healthy Eating for Life to Prevent and Treat Diabetes, PCRM with Patricia Bertron, R.D.

Nutrition Guide for Clinicians, Physicians Committee for Responsible Medicine

Plant Roots, Rex Bowlby

Becoming Whole: The Story of My Complete Recovery from Breast Cancer, Meg Wolff

Find Awesome Animal-Free Restaurants
www.happycow.net
www.vegdining.com
www.vrg.org/travel/index.htm

Information On Buying Clubs
Groups of individuals band together to buy from wholesalers in large quantities. You can join an existing group in your area or start your own, ordering bulk foods in 25 pound lots. Here are some of the wholesalers.

Associated Buyers
  www.assocbuyers.com

Azure Standard
  www.azurestandard.com

Neshaminy Valley
  www.nvorganic.com

United Buying Clubs
  www.unitedbuyingclubs.com

Information On Banishing Toxic Chemicals From Your Life

Environmental Working Group
www.ewg.org

Organic Consumers Association
www.organicconsumers.org

Silent Spring Institute
www.silentspring.org

Susan Jeske (former Ms. America harmed by toxic personal care products)
www.susanjeske.com (click on the toxic cosmetics link)

Climate Destabilization

Stop Global Warming
www.biteglobalwarming.org

Livestock's Long Shadow—free download of United Nations report
www.fao.org/docrep/010/a0701e/a0701e00.htm

Other Next Steps

Star athlete Ruth Heidrich, Ph.D.
www.ruthheidrich.com

Weightlifting and exercise
www.joycevedral.com
www.organic-athlete.com
http://veganbodybuilding.com

Organic gardening
www.vegsource.com/gardening

The Plight Of Farmed And Other Animals

FARM
www.farmusa.org

United Poultry Concerns
www.upc-online.org

Compassion over Killing
www.cok.net

Humane Society of the United States
http://humanesociety.org

In Defense of Animals
http://www.idausa.org

Farm Sanctuary
www.farmsanctuary.org

Tribe of Heart
http://tribeofheart.org

Howard Lyman, the cattle rancher who stopped eating meat
http://madcowboy.com

So-called "humane" meat
www.humanemyth.org

PETA
www.peta.org

Fishing Hurts
http://fishinghurts.com

Dire threats to life in the oceans
www.sharkwater.com

Defenders of Wildlife
http://defenders.org

Animals Asia
  www.animalsasia.org

Best Friends (mostly companion animals)
  http://bestfriends.org

Dakota: A Novel, Martha Grimes

The Face on Your Plate: The Truth About Food, Jeffrey Masson

The Politics Of Food, Medicine, Household Chemicals, And Tobacco

You probably don't believe that the USDA, the FDA, or any other government agency is genuinely and effectively looking out for your best interests. Nonetheless, you may be surprised to understand how much profit there is in poor health.

Food Politics, Marion Nestle

Appetite for Profit, Michele Simon

Overdosed America, John Abramson, M.D.

The Cigarette Century, Allan M. Brandt

The Hundred Year Lie, Randall Fitzgerald

Alternative Medicine

National Center for Complementary and Alternative Medicine
  http://nccam.nih.gov

Guided imagery information and programs
  www.thehealingmind.org

Benson-Henry Institute for Mind Body Medicine
  www.mbmi.org

Mindfulness meditation
  http://www.mindfulnesscds.com

Videos On DVD

The Witness

Peaceable Kingdom

Stopping Cancer Before It Starts (Michael Greger, M.D.)

Super Size Me

Food Inc.

Sharkwater *(should stop you cold from ever being tempted to eat fish)*

Any videos from Dr. John McDougall (*www.drmcdougall.com*) or watch Star McDougallers on his website

Eating

Macro for the Mainstream

Eating Right for Cancer Survival

Behind the Mask

Earthlings

Magazines

Veg News
www.vegnews.com

Vegan Voice
http://veganic.net

Finding Peer Review Articles

Search peer reviewed journals from around the world at this site maintained by the U.S. National Library of Medicine and the National Institutes of Health.
www.ncbi.nlm.nih.gov/pubmed

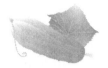

References

To keep this book affordable and save a lot of trees, references are posted at *www.perfectformuladiet.com* instead of being included in this book. I studied more than a thousand references to put together the ideas and information in this book. You can download all the top studies that I directly used in each chapter on the website.

If you want to check out the sources yourself—which I strongly encourage—it will also be easy to bring the reference list from the website to your local or online library.

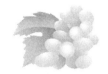

Index

Acupuncture, 226–228

Addiction, 27, 107

Advanced glycation end products (AGEs), 187, 193, 198

Affirmations, 102–103

Aging, 2, 67, 161–162, 167, 182, 184, 187–188

Air pollution, 94, 206–207, 209, 235

Alcohol, 89, 136, 224

Allergy, 23, 42, 84, 148, 161, 169, 174, 191, 200, 202, 213, 232

Alzheimer's disease, 77, 140, 142, 148, 150, 161–164, 167, 193, 202

American Institute for Cancer Research, 90

Amino acids, 32–42, 45–49, 54, 173, 182, 184, 186, 194, 239

Antioxidants, 78, 83, 135, 188, 190, 198

Apoptosis, 4, 183

Arachidonic acid, 187, 191

Arthritis, 137, 141–142, 146, 149, 153, 161–163, 167, 173–174, 176, 188, 191, 193, 209, 221, 223

Artificial sweeteners, 26, 55–56, 89

Asthma, 20, 132, 142, 148–149,161, 169, 174, 183, 211, 213–214, 221, 223, 232

Athletes, 47–50, 57, 249

Autism, 161,205, 211

Autoimmune disease, 148, 161, 169, 173, 177, 179, 200, 223

Bacteria, 33–34, 42, 52, 79, 91, 154, 172, 175, 182, 196, 213

Barnard, Dr. Neal, xiv, 245, 247

Binge eating, xi, xii, 108

Bioaccumulation, 201

Biofeedback, 226

Body mass index (BMI)
  Definition, 13
  Optimal range, 13, 21, 145

Bone health, 77–78, 142, 149, 162, 194–198, 220

Breast milk, 38, 44, 201, 203

Budgeting, 127–130

Cachexia, 42, 184

Calcium, 6, 57, 59, 77, 132, 135, 171, 194–197

Campbell, Dr. T. Colin, xiv, 133–135, 142, 247

Cancer, 13, 20, 26, 42–43, 46, 52–53, 77–78, 84, 86, 90, 131–132, 136, 139, 141–142, 148, 152, 161–164, 167, 182–184, 189, 191–193, 197–198, 200, 202, 205, 210–211, 213, 252
  Bladder, 140
  Breast, 52, 79, 134–135, 137–139, 141–142, 164, 182–183, 192, 248
  Colon, 135–136, 139, 163–164, 182, 194
  Endometrial, 140–141, 150, 192
  Leukemia, 135
  Liver, 140, 182, 203
  Lung, 135, 137, 164, 182
  Non-Hodgkins lymphoma, 74, 134
  Ovarian, 50, 138, 140–141, 182, 192
  Pancreatic, 137, 149, 182
  Prostate, 90, 136–139, 141, 143, 164, 183, 192

  Skin, 164
  Stomach, 164, 182
  Testicular, 138–139, 192, 205

Cardiovascular disease, 52, 77, 84, 136, 142, 149–150, 152–153, 161–162, 164, 167, 171, 183, 187, 191, 193, 202, 206, 221, 223–224, 227

Celiac disease, 83

Centenarians, 162

China Study, 133–135, 144, 247

Chiropractic, 226

Chocolate, 52, 86–87, 89, 94–95, 229, 246

Cleaning products, 93, 155, 178, 209, 211–217, 243, 245

Climate change — see climate destabilization

Climate destabilization 203, 229–238, 240, 249

Coffee, 88–89, 94, 121

Collagen, 31, 173

Cost of food — see budgeting

Cost of health care, 147–148

Counseling, 12, 95, 223, 228

Cravings, xiv, 5, 12, 20, 23–25, 27, 29, 59, 67–68, 70–71, 75, 78, 80, 82, 92, 108, 116

C reactive protein (CRP), 143, 156–157, 162–164, 166, 175–177, 219, 224

Depression, 53, 148, 161, 163, 189, 223

Detoxification, 20–21, 52, 72, 86, 93, 96, 101, 107, 203, 207, 217, 228

Diabetes, 17–18, 60, 74, 77, 79, 84–85, 135, 137, 141–142, 148–149, 150, 152–153, 161, 163, 167, 173, 183, 193, 200, 202, 205, 221–222, 247–248

Drought, 231–232, 236, 238

Eating disorders, 95, 108

Energy density, 19, 80

Environmental Working Group, 212, 249

Epidemiology, 133, 137, 139, 143

Estrogen, 52, 78, 140, 182, 187, 192–193, 198, 200, 205, 213, 240

Exercise, 12, 15, 21, 47–48, 92, 94, 134, 136, 219–221, 224, 226, 228, 240, 249

Extinction, 190, 204, 240

Farmers markets, 114, 122, 128, 245, 246

Fiber, 18–19, 59, 72–73, 75–76, 78, 82, 177, 189, 203

Fish oil, 54–55, 190, 198, 246

Flame retardant — see PDBE

Flavonoids, 52

Flax seed, 54, 63, 69, 85, 92, 114, 128, 142–143, 189–190, 198

Flu, 151–152

Fluoride, 195

Forests, 231, 234–235

Fragrance, 209, 212–214, 216

Fuhrman, Dr. Joel, xiv, 246–247

Fungus, 175

Galactose, 50

Genetically modified "food," 26

Genetics, 7–9, 35, 162, 173

Global warming — see climate destabilization

Gluten, 83–84

Glycemic index, 59

Green spaces, 223–224, 226, 228

Greger, Dr. Michael, xiv, 246–247, 252

Growth factor — see IGF-1

Guided imagery, 223, 226, 228, 251

Gum disease — see periodontitis

Heavy metals, 210–205, 207

Heidrich, Dr. Ruth, 50, 246–247, 249

Heterocyclic amines, 187, 193–194

High blood pressure, 16, 60, 77, 79, 137, 143, 146, 149–150, 152, 161, 163, 193, 202, 222, 227

Hormone disruption, 199, 206, 210, 215

Hydrogenated vegetable oil — see trans-fatty acids

IGF-1, 181–186, 197, 240

Immune system, 4, 42, 93–94, 154, 156, 160, 169, 172–175, 178–190, 197, 200, 205, 211, 220–221, 223, 227
    Balance of, 52
    Response to foreign protein, 41, 46, 172–173, 175, 177

Indoor pollution, 209, 211

Inflammation, 19, 42, 52, 86, 142, 153, 159, 163–165, 169, 180, 181, 183, 186–188, 196–197, 210, 220–223, 227–228
    Acute, 157, 166
    Causes of, 154–155, 172, 176, 178, 189, 206, 214, 219, 224
    Chronic, 151–152, 157–158, 161–162, 166–167, 170–175, 177, 179, 182–185, 240
    Definition, 153
    Functions of, 153–156, 160, 166
    Measurement of, 156–157

Inflammator, 154–158, 160, 165–167, 169, 172, 178–179, 180, 182, 204, 206–207, 210, 215, 217, 221

Insulin, 19, 60, 78, 83–84, 93, 142, 182, 186, 198, 222

Interleukin-6 (IL-6), 143, 156–157, 162–163, 166, 220

Iron, 57, 59, 188, 212

Isoflavones, 52, 78

Juice, 75, 88–89, 92, 116, 243

Kidneys, 40, 42–43, 46, 78, 148, 150, 174, 178, 184, 193

Kwashiorkor, 45

Labels, 82, 87, 92, 115, 191, 212, 214, 216, 245–246

Lactose, 50–51, 140

Leaky gut, 42, 175

Lignans, 52, 54

Liver, 20, 39–40, 46, 72, 83, 93, 181

Marasmus, 45

Marine algae, 54, 190, 246

McDougall, Dr. John, xiv, 243–244, 246–247, 252

McDougall, Mary, 243–244

Meal plans — see not-meal plans

Meditation, 219, 223, 226, 251

Mercury and fish, 141, 203, 205

Millward, Dr. D. Joe, 47

Minerals, 4, 33, 45, 51, 57–58, 67, 71, 77–78, 80, 82–83, 90–91, 100, 129, 142, 194–196, 227

Molecular mimicry, 173

Multimorbidity, 146–147, 161

Musk, 213

Natural food stores, 60, 114, 122, 128, 245

Nitrogen, 32–33, 39–40

Not-meal plans, 63–66, 240, 244

Obesity, 7–8, 46, 67, 77–78, 132, 134, 144, 183, 202

Olive oil, 6, 11, 85

Omega-3 fatty acids, 53–55, 63, 85, 176, 187, 189–190, 198, 246

Omega-6 fatty acids, 26, 53–55, 58, 63, 85, 187, 189–191

Organic Consumers Association, 212, 249

Osteoporosis — see bone health

Oxidation, 187–188, 190, 198

Paget's disease, 195

Parabens, 213

Parkinson's disease, 140–141, 150, 200, 202

PDBE, 202–203

Periodontitis, 148, 161, 196–197, 223

Persistent organic pollutants, 200–210, 213

Personal care products, 93, 178, 209, 211, 213, 215–216, 240, 249

Pesticides, 93, 200–201, 203, 205, 207, 213, 234, 236

PFOA, 210

Phthalates, 213

Physicians Committee for Responsible Medicine (PCRM), 60, 246

Phytochemicals, 51–52, 54, 58, 63, 70–73, 75–78, 82, 90–91, 96, 129, 178, 188–189

Plaque, 84, 170–172, 179, 183

Prematurity, 148–150, 161, 205

Pritikin Diet, 177

Progesterone, 192

Protein, 4, 11–12, 21, 31, 40, 44, 46, 48–59, 78, 83, 92, 100, 107, 121, 134–135, 139–141, 155, 166, 169–170, 172–186, 188, 196–198, 235, 239–240
    Deficiency diseases, 45
    Digestion of, 41–43
    Discovery of, 31
    Function of, 31, 47, 194
    Human protein requirements, 37–39, 41, 44, 47–48
    Powder, 25, 90
    Storage, 35–36
    Structure, 32–35
    Weight gain and, 14, 18, 44–45

Purpose in life, 230, 236

Rebound effect, 159, 164

Recipes, 118, 124, 243–245

Risk factors, 84, 103, 134, 138, 146, 152

Seventh Day Adventist, 15–16, 85, 133, 136–137, 144

Sleep, 219, 221–222, 225–226, 228, 240

Smoking, 94, 149, 152, 155, 205, 224, 226, 228

Soda, 26, 88, 90, 114, 123

Stages of change, 105–106

Statistics, 132

Steroids, 192

Storms, 231

Stress, 42, 64–65, 99, 106, 153, 223–224, 226–228

Superfood, 6–7, 9, 239

Supplements, 47, 52, 54, 90–93, 129–130, 184, 188, 190, 195, 198, 246

Tea, 52, 88–89, 94, 121–122, 136

Topsoil, 235

Traditions, 124

Trans-fatty acids (hydrogenated vegetable oil), 26, 55, 83, 87, 90, 115, 123, 176, 191

Triclosan, 213

Troubleshooting, 91–95

Vegetable oil, 25–26, 53, 55, 58, 63, 66, 79–80, 83, 85, 90, 115–119, 122, 128, 135, 138, 189–191, 243

Vitamin B12, 91, 129

Vitamin D, 91, 129, 195–196

Water pollution, 203, 235–236

Water scarcity, 235

World Cancer Research Fund, 90, 157

World Health Organization, 37, 232

Wrinkles, 188, 198, 214

Workplace, 120, 215, 229, 232

Yoga, 223, 226

Who Else Can Benefit From
The Perfect Formula Diet?

Order another copy for someone you care about online at
www.perfectformuladiet.com or at an online bookstore. Shop these
sites for the best price and to pay by credit card.

Or, for your convenience, you can order direct from the publisher
with this form.

Quantity	Price	Total
_____ *The Perfect Formula Diet*	$18.95 (each book)	$ _____

Shipping and Handling: $3 for the first book and $1 more for
each additional book for U.S. priority mail within the U.S. $ _____

Grand total $ _____

☐ Check or money order enclosed (made payable to *Perfect Planet Solutions*)

Book recipient:

Name: _____

Address: _____

_____

Your phone number (to be used only for questions on your order): _____

Your email address (to be used only for questions on your order):_____

Comments: _____

_____

_____

Contact *info@perfectformuladiet.com* with any questions

Mail this form with check or money order payment to:

Perfect Planet Solutions
5580 La Jolla Blvd #459
La Jolla, CA 92037

THANK YOU!

LaVergne, TN USA
30 December 2009

168506LV00010B/128/P

9 780984 106738